W9-CFL-598

The Vitamin Sourcebook

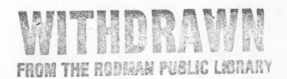
WITHDRAWN
FROM THE RODMAN PUBLIC LIBRARY

The Vitamin Sourcebook

by

Tonia Reinhard, M.S., R.D.

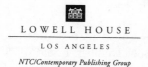

LOWELL HOUSE

LOS ANGELES

NTC/Contemporary Publishing Group

RODMAN PUBLIC LIBRARY

3821200283274
Main Adult
612.399 R369
Reinhard, Tonia
The vitamin sourcebook

Library of Congress Cataloging-in-Publication Data

Reinhard, Tonia.
    The vitamin sourcebook / by Tonia Reinhard.
      p. cm.
    Includes bibliographical references and index.
    ISBN 1-56565-878-7
    1. Vitamins in human nutrition. 2. Vitamins. I. Title.
  QP771.R45 1998
  612.3'99—dc21   98-34410
                                              CIP

Published by Lowell House, a division of NTC/Contemporary Publishing
Group, Inc. 4255 West Touhy Avenue, Lincolnwood, Illinois 60646-1975 U.S.A.

Copyright © 1998 by NTC/Contemporary Publishing Group.
All rights reserved. No part of this work may be reproduced, stored
in a retrieval system, or transmitted in any form or by any means
electronic, mechanical, photocopying, recording, or otherwise without
prior permission of NTC/Contemporary Publishing Group, Inc.

Requests for such permissions should be addressed to:
Lowell House
2020 Avenue of the Stars, Suite 300
Los Angeles, CA 90067

Design by Andrea Reider
Illustrations by Eve Guianan

Printed and bound in the United States of America
International Standard Book Number: 1-56565-878-7
10 9 8 7 6 5 4 3 2 1

*To John, Faye, and Brendan for patience when fingers were
glued to the keyboard not doing anything else, and for generating
laughter to keep us all going; and to Gea DeRubeis-Pacifico,
Guy Pacifico, Lita and Marcus Badia, and Sandra Manzo for
support and doses of reality that reined in long discourses on
the merits of tofu.*

Acknowledgments

Thanks to Lynn Kuligowski, R.D., an extraordinary dietitian, for help with research; Soraya Issa, R.D., my other sister, for help in reviewing the stuff and sprinkling inspiration along the way; David Klurfeld, department chair and general brilliant thinker; and the Captain, Paula Kirk-Labadie, who started it all.

Contents

List of Tables

List of Figures

Introduction

A young, vibrant blond raised her hand before the question had barely escaped my lips, as if she were reaching for the buzzer on a TV game show. It was always the first query of many I would ask the college students in my "Intro Nutrition 101" class during the first lecture: "What is the most important nutrition question that you expect to be answered by the end of this semester?"

With an earnest expression usually indicative of the most diligent students, she asked, "Which vitamins should I be taking to be healthy?"

In a sense, her question is paradoxically the easiest and toughest to answer. Textbooks and popular books are filled with descriptions of vitamins and laundry lists of their food sources. At the same time, researchers grapple with the complexities of these tiny compounds in numerous studies—most of which are trying to prove or disprove whether vitamins can do more than simply prevent vitamin deficiencies. Doing more means preventing a host of diseases that plague us. The list of diseases which scientists are now studying as having links to vitamins seems to grow longer with each edition of the daily newspaper, and usually heart disease and cancer are at the forefront. There are several reasons for these two killers heading the list: together, heart disease and cancer account for 75 percent of deaths each year in the United States, or 1.5 million people.

But college nutrition students tend to be more interested in enhancing their current health and physical performance, whether they're into bodybuilding or trying to boost their immune systems so they don't get sick, and less so with the concerns of middle age, such as high cholesterol and blood pressure. These last two problems, and a few more, such as diabetes and weight control, are the common ones that I faced along with the clients who brought them to nutrition counseling sessions. But regardless of our age and our reasons, most of us share more than a passing interest in nutrition—we share a fundamental belief that the food choices we make on a daily basis affect our health.

Some might say that this kind of thinking is a recent development, but they would be wrong. Huang Ti, the Yellow Emperor of China in the eighth century B.C.E., wrote, "Hence, if too much salt is eaten, the pulse hardens," foreshadowing our current understanding of salt's effect on blood pressure. Medical history shows us that the ancients from many civilizations linked various diseases to one's diet, albeit erroneously in many cases. But the fast-paced lifestyle which has come to define the so-called modern age ignored wisdom from the past in its pursuit of fast meals and quick health fixes. It probably took millions of angioplasties and coronary bypass surgeries to remind us that preventing a problem is a lot better than trying to fix the problem later. That's not to say that modern techniques such as these have not saved countless lives, but the focus on prevention will probably save lives, too, and hopefully, in a less painful and costly way.

Most nutrition professionals would agree that the field hit the big time with the 1988 U.S. Surgeon General's Report on Nutrition and Health:

> For the two out of three Americans who do not smoke and do not drink excessively, one personal choice seems to influence long-term health prospects more than any other: what we eat.

That statement continues to resonate into our decade, based on available scientific research, but the focus has shifted away from reducing dietary intake of constituents in foods thought to negatively impact health, such as fat, to ensuring optimal intake of others, such as antioxidant vitamins, that do the opposite.

In writing this book, my hope is to provide a user-friendly approach to understanding what we know vitamins can do, and what we think they can't do, in a practical guide that helps you to put it all together at each meal. And remember one important point—one of the Japanese Dietary Guidelines says it best: "Enjoy every meal you eat."

How to Use This Book

To help make the most of the information in this book, consider completing the diet questionnaires included at the end of Chapter 1. Your answers will help you determine if your diet provides optimal amounts of each of the vitamins that are discussed in subsequent chapters.

In addition, each chapter includes:

1. "Where to Find the Vitamin" tables showing food sources of each vitamin and the amount they contain and how each source stacks up to the daily recommended amount.
2. "Great Diet Ideas for the Vitamin" sidebars with practical tips showing you how to boost the amount of each vitamin in your diet.
3. "Four-Star Foods" sidebars listing four top foods for each vitamin.
4. "Check Your Diet for the Vitamin" quizzes to rate your diet for each vitamin and compare your intake to current recommendations for each one.

The Vitamin Sourcebook

Jump Start:
A Nutrition Primer

Because we all eat several times a day, this simple act confers the status of food expert on us all. Ostensibly by association, everyone becomes an expert in nutrition as well. This is alright most of the time, especially if it leads people to think for themselves and become more aware of the importance of nutrition. Two articles in my local paper within a week of each other, however, sounded a warning siren.

The first item, in the business section, spotlighted a prosperous fellow who owns several health food stores. He proudly declared that, in addition to being financially successful, he has personally interviewed over 100,000 people in his stores. By virtue of this, and years of dispensing vitamin supplement recommendations along with diet advice, he lists his profession as "nutrition counselor." That story reinforces the problem of untrained, noncredentialed individuals dispensing health advice, in particular those who have an inherent conflict of interest because their livelihood depends on selling products.

The other news item had more serious and immediate consequences. An osteopathic doctor practicing in West Michigan injected one of his patients with a dose of essiac, a popular herbal brew. As the compound circulated in the patient's blood, she complained of thirst, chills, and a severe headache, while a vivid blue line appeared along the top of her forehead. By that evening, she was dead of multiple organ system failure in the emergency room of the local hospital.

On the surface, the two stories may seem unrelated, but in both cases, someone was taking on a role best left to an expert; a dietitian is the right choice for counseling people on diets, and the osteopath should have consulted with a toxicologist before trying an unorthodox treatment. Both scenarios highlight the problem of promoting unproven, and possibly dangerous, therapies.

In some ways, the science of nutrition has brought these problems on itself. Consumers are assaulted by a constant barrage of conflicting reports on diet and health, leading many to throw their hands up in disgust and lament, "everything causes cancer!" What isn't conveyed by media reports is that nutrition is a young science, with the discovery of the vitamins heralding its birth back in the late 1800s. But it is a science and, as such, relies on the scientific method to make new discoveries. The very nature of the scientific method, which consists of repeated experiments and reproducibility of results, raises conflicts, just as it should!

This section introduces nutrition and its basic concepts, laying the groundwork for an understanding of how the star performers of the nutrition scene, the vitamins, fit into the intricate mosaic of human health.

Chapter **One**

Let's Talk Nutrition: The Six Essential Nutrients

A framework for understanding vitamins starts with a definition of the umbrella under which these vital compounds are but one piece of the puzzle—nutrition. Any number of textbooks can provide a working definition, some more inclusive than others, but most would agree on that provided by the Council on Food and Nutrition of the American Medical Association:

> Nutrition is the science of food, the nutrients, and the substances therein, their action, interaction, and balance in relation to health and disease, and the process by which the organism ingests, digests, absorbs, transports, utilizes, and excretes food substances.

Quite a mouthful, and if you haven't guessed, we are the organisms in question, along with any other species on earth that biologists consider to be alive. That definition is good for showing the scope of the science of nutrition, but it leaves out the more human factor of food behavior. And it is food behavior, or the food choices we make on a daily basis and why we make them, which determines

3

how nutrition affects our health. Another way to say this is, once we know which foods and in what amounts are beneficial to our health, why don't we eat those foods in those amounts?

Of course that's the proverbial million-dollar question, and it doesn't lend itself to easy answers. Cynics might respond that humans are inherently lazy and hedonistic, seeking after pleasure first and foremost. While that may explain it for some of us, a more enlightened response would be that our food behavior is influenced by culture, beliefs, heritage, socioeconomic status, lifestyle, and a host of other equally important factors. It's no surprise, then, that simply knowing which foods are more health promoting doesn't mean people actually eat those foods. But awareness is the first step, and only after acquiring correct information can a person choose to change his or her behavior.

A growing number of people are frustrated by what they perceive as conflicting information. Nutrition is a young science compared to other scientific disciplines, which means that nutrition studies got a late start and have continued to boom in the past few decades. In addition, as new reports came out, other researchers followed the scientific method and tried to repeat the same experiments. If the results of a study can be reproduced in similar studies, the conclusions are more reliable.

A good example is the recent flap about beta-carotene and lung cancer. Many studies have shown that people who eat lots of fruits and vegetables had lower rates of several different types of cancer (among these, lung cancer). Trying to figure out just what it is in fruits and vegetables producing the beneficial effect, however, is fairly complicated. Some subsequent studies have suggested that beta-carotene was the likely magic bullet, and researchers designed a special type of study to test that theory.

What they found was that smokers who took beta-carotene supplements actually had a higher risk for lung cancer! Since then, another study showed the same results. While even more studies would really convince everyone, the fact that the first results were reproduced in another study would suggest that smokers should avoid taking beta-carotene supplements. A look at the different types of studies that nutrition researchers do will help explain another reason for sometimes conflicting reports on diet and health, and will also prepare you for the upcoming chapters on vitamins, which focus on the latest research.

Why a Rat and Not a Person?

Another reason for the seeming contradictions in new nutrition information has to do with the different types of studies and the fact that the media tend to report results as soon as they are published, sometimes sooner. Because of this, no filtering occurs, which might help to put each single study in a broader context of what has come before and how to interpret the results. Research results can be difficult for experts to decipher, let alone a newspaper reporter who has no background in science. Yet this is how most Americans come by their nutrition information. Little wonder that each new report seems to add to consumer confusion instead of resolving it.

Scientists use four basic types of studies, each with its own strengths and weaknesses, to either prove or disprove a hypothesis, or a guess they may have about something (see Table 1.1). The first, and most familiar, is the laboratory study, which can include animals or simply test tubes. Lab studies can provide details on why a specific effect occurs, such as how vitamin C boosts immune function. One reason for doing this is that animals can be dissected after the study, in sharp contrast to human subjects.

Laboratory Study

Another strength of a lab study is the control that the researchers have over their experiments. They can use a specific breed of rat, knowing all the physiologic background of the strain, and are assured that all subjects will be extremely similar. In contrast, a group of seemingly similar humans presents many more variables than 100 "Sprague Dawley" rats! Finally, researchers can use as many rats or rabbits as they can afford, and the greater the number of subjects, the more valid the results.

The major weakness of lab studies is obvious, however; just because a study works a certain way in a rat doesn't mean the same applies to a human being. When the media report the latest research results, people often do not pay attention to the fact that it was an animal study and that applicability to humans remains to be proven. In addition, researchers have to be on their toes to use an appropriate animal model in a particular study because different species vary in how similar they are to humans with regard to a specific function. As an example, ferrets are the best animal for studying the absorption of beta-carotene, since their physiology most closely resembles humans in this regard.

Case Study

This type of study focuses on one individual, usually someone who has exhibited an interesting trait. A somewhat recent example comes to mind: a few years back, the *New England Journal of Medicine* reported that a man in his nineties, who had been eating an average of a dozen eggs a week, had the blood cholesterol levels of a healthy teenager. This obviously surprised his physician and countless nutrition professionals who read the published report, because age and male gender are both risk factors for high cholesterol. To add a dozen eggs a week, which conventional wisdom of the time implicated as raising blood cholesterol, was unthinkable! While these reports are intriguing and can lead to further research, the effect of diet on one individual is not significant.

Epidemiologic Study

So if one person isn't enough, what about an entire population? Epidemiologic, or population, studies compare disease rates among groups of people around the world, and look for correlations between disease and dietary habits. It was this type of study that led researchers to the association between a Mediterranean-type diet and a lower risk for heart disease. Epidemiologic studies are useful in pointing to a possible connection between diet and disease, laying the groundwork for further studies. Unfortunately, these studies can only show a statistical association, but not cause and effect. In other words, just because a study reports that people who eat a high-fiber diet tend to get colon cancer less often, the study doesn't prove that dietary fiber prevents the disease. It might just be that something else about the high-fiber diet, or the kind of people who eat that way, is protecting against colon cancer.

Intervention/Clinical Trial Study

An intervention study compares the effects of a treatment, or intervention, on a group of people or subjects, called the experimental group, to another group, who received no treatment, called the controls. The control group is sometimes called the placebo group, which simply means that they received a fake treatment or "sugar pill" instead of the real treatment. The intervention study is by far the most powerful of all research designs because it demonstrates the effect of a given treatment. Recent examples include the Physicians' Health Study, which proved that a small daily dose of aspirin reduced the risk for heart attack in men.

So if this type of study is so good, why isn't it used all the time? It's very expensive to conduct clinical trials, partly because humans are involved, requiring longer periods of time for treatment than animal subjects. In addition, blood draws and other assessment methods require trained personnel, which adds to the cost. But even with powerful intervention studies, the results are only as good as another study's ability to duplicate the results.

TABLE 1.1   Pros and Cons of Different Types of Studies

Study Type	What Is It?	Pro	Con
Laboratory	animal studies	similarity of subjects	an animal is not a person, so results can't be applied; can use numerous subjects
		can dissect subjects to learn more	
		usually short duration (based on life span of animal)	
	in vitro don't use a living organism; use tissues, or chemical experiment	inexpensive short duration	less validity because not in a living organism
Case study	follows the clinical course of one person	human study; more valid than animal or in vitro	less validity because only one person observed
Epidemiologic	compares populations of people with regard to disease incidence and some aspect of diet	large numbers; more valid	can't show cause and effect, only statistical correlation
Intervention/ Clinical trial	human study comparing the effects of a treatment to no treatment or a different treatment	good validity; applicability to other people	very expensive

Note: Even the best results of any type of study must be reproduced by other studies before they can be considered valid.

The Last Word?

The next time a news headline screams, "Broccoli Causes Cancer!" take a few minutes to evaluate the study. Look at a few simple criteria, such as whether it was a human or animal study. If it was a human study, how many people participated? Was it an intervention study or an epidemiologic study? And finally, if the results contradict research that has preceded this study, remember that reproducibility of those results will be necessary before taking the information too seriously. Researchers are just doing their job by continually asking questions; generally, they end up with many more questions after doing a study than answers to the first question they asked. Smart consumers will wait before acting on the results of a new study.

Six, Count 'Em: The Essential Nutrients

Nutrition concerns itself with the study of foods and the numerous compounds they contain. However, some preferential treatment is in order for the essential nutrients. The word *essential* refers to the fact that we have to ingest these compounds through our diet; our body can't make them. We need these substances to grow and maintain our bodies. Adults don't tend to grow as do infants and children, but they still need to repair and replace body tissues.

As an example, red blood cells have a limited life span of four months. After that time, the body has to make new ones. To do that, it needs specific nutrients. You might consider nutrients to be building blocks for all forms of life. In some ways, we are not too different from an ear of corn or a bowl of rice (see Fig. 1.1). Although the comparison isn't exactly flattering, it illustrates that the human body is made up of similar components as the foods we eat, which is why those foods are nutritious to us!

The six essential nutrient groups which we must obtain through our diet are water, carbohydrate, fat, protein, minerals, and vitamins (see Table 1.2). Within each group, we need several nutrients. For example, we need thirteen vitamins and fifteen minerals. Water is

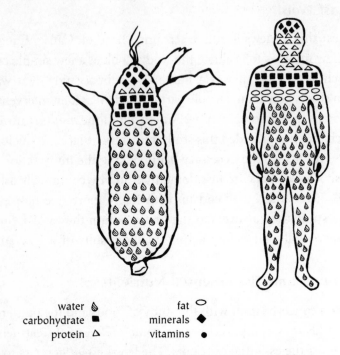

water	◊	fat	○
carbohydrate	■	minerals	◆
protein	△	vitamins	●

FIGURE 1.1   **Body Composition of Human Versus Plant**

by far the most vital: you can get by without vitamin C for a few months, but a shortage of water will be life threatening within days. This is generally true for all the nutrients, with a deficiency of some adversely affecting us sooner than others. Another important principle is that only fat, carbohydrate, and protein provide energy in the form of calories. Each of the billion cells in our bodies is a small microcosm of the whole, and while each needs all the essential nutrients, the most critical in the short term are water and energy.

Each essential nutrient has a particular function in the body which can't be performed by any other nutrient. Overall, water, vitamins, and minerals help convert the energy nutrients, fat, carbohydrate, and protein into energy the body can use. Aside from the obvious need for energy to fuel our physical activity, the body uses energy to build and

TABLE 1.2   The Six Essential Nutrient Groups

	Made Up of	Names of Nutrients in the Group
Carbohydrate	Carbon, Hydrogen, Oxygen	Starch, simple sugars to yield glucose
Fat (Lipids)	Carbon, Hydrogen, Oxygen	2 essential fatty acids: Linoleic, Linolenic
Protein	Carbon, Hydrogen, Oxygen, Nitrogen	9 essential amino acids
Vitamins	Carbon, Hydrogen, Oxygen, Nitrogen (some contain minerals)	A, D, E, K, C, Thiamin, Niacin, Riboflavin, Cobalamine, Pyridoxine, Folate, Biotin, Pantothenic Acid, Choline
Minerals	Basic elements	Calcium, Chloride, Chromium, Copper, Fluoride, Iodine, Iron, Magnesium, Manganese, Molybdenum, Phosphorus, Potassium, Selenium, Sodium, Sulfur, Zinc
Water	Hydrogen, Oxygen	Simply water!

maintain its components such as muscle, bone, and blood. A chemist once described the human body as a mini-chemistry lab forced to conduct millions of chemical reactions every day. A fairly apt metaphor, and the vitamins are among the industrious little chemists working to change the food we eat into fuel, glue, bricks, and other building materials to keep the main building in good repair.

Quick Notes on Each Nutrient Group

This book, and especially the next three sections, focuses on vitamins, but a quick summary of each essential nutrient group's functions is in order.

Carbohydrates

Although this group has sometimes gotten a bad rap, it includes a variety of compounds which have implications for health, with the basic function of providing energy for the body's needs. Our main source is green plants, which convert water and carbon dioxide in the air to carbohydrate, with the help of sunlight and chlorophyll. Carbohydrates are either simple or complex, with simple carbohydrates consisting of sugars. The most common form of sugar, glucose, is the energy currency that travels in our blood to keep the cells fed.

Complex carbohydrate refers to starch and fiber, and of the two, humans can only digest and derive energy from starch. Although we don't have the needed enzymes to break down fiber, it helps the body in other ways. The fact that we can't break it down means that it keeps moving along the intestinal tract, stimulating bowel function and keeping it healthy. There is good evidence that a high-fiber diet can lower the risk for colon cancer. Friendly bacteria that live in the colon can break it down, and the by-products appear to have a healthful effect on colon function and in lowering cholesterol.

You can see that the bad rap is undeserved: far from being "fattening" additions to the diet, a generous intake of complex carbohydrate may actually help with weight control by replacing higher-calorie fats. Aside from its potential health benefits, fiber also makes a person feel full (called satiety), which may reduce calorie intake. The key is to emphasize complex carbohydrates, and use sugars only moderately. And finally, complex carbohydrates are one of the best ways to obtain the B vitamins, with whole grains being an excellent source.

How much is the right amount? That depends on you and your total energy needs in a day. Remember, the type of carbohydrate is everything. Load up on food sources such as fruits, vegetables, whole grain breads, cereals, and other grain products. Cut back on sources which are mainly desserts such as cookies, cakes, pies, candy, and sweetened drinks. To ensure that you get enough fiber in your diet, you might even consider limiting your intake of added sugars and processed grain products that offer no fiber. These include white bread, presweetened cereals, and crackers, muffins, and bagels that are not whole grain. Shoot for 50 to 60 percent of your total calories to eat as carbohydrates. If your daily calorie intake is around 2,000, you should take in slightly more than half, or 1,000 calories, as carbs. Table 1.3 illustrates a healthy example focusing on carbohydrate choices.

Fat

Most people think of fat as something to avoid in their daily diets to prevent heart attacks and keep from becoming obese. But as with carbohydrate, the reputation is largely undeserved, with different types of fat serving many vital roles in the body. The type of fat we

TABLE 1.3 **Carbohydrate in a Sample Menu**

Meal	Foods	Amount	Carb (g)	Fiber (g)
Breakfast	whole grain cereal (such as Shredded Wheat)	1 cup	30	4
	orange juice	1 cup	30	1
	banana	1 medium	30	2
Lunch	whole wheat bread	2 slices	30	4
	apple	1 medium	30	4
	baby carrots, raw	2 ounces	10	2
Dinner	vegetable stir-fry (red pepper, onion, broccoli)	2 cups	15	7
	rice	1 cup	55	1
	romaine lettuce and tomato salad	1 cup	5	2
Snack	graham crackers	6	30	1
	crunchy peanut butter	2 tablespoons	7	3
Total			272	31

carry on our bodies, triglyceride, is the same type we eat in foods. While we may complain about how fat we are, if we had to store our energy reserves as carbohydrate, we'd be huge! Fat takes up roughly half the space, in chemical terms, as carbohydrate. The reason for fat being the perfect form of reserve energy in the body actually accounts for its higher calorie value—9 calories per gram, compared to carbohydrate and protein at 4 calories per gram.

Fat is also useful as an insulator against temperature extremes, and it protects vital organs by cushioning them. On a smaller scale, fat molecules make up the protective membranes surrounding individual body cells and other important structures. The fat in foods adds to flavor, texture, and "mouth feel," which is a food technologist's term to describe the creamy sensation in your mouth when you eat a food containing fat. Fat also contributes to a feeling of satiety, a feeling of fullness after a meal. This may be one reason why people who dramatically cut back on their fat intake can't seem to get enough food.

Getting back to vitamins, several of them require the presence of fat in foods to be properly absorbed and used by the body. Some people who have conditions causing difficulty in fat absorption end up becoming deficient in the fat soluble vitamins (those requiring fat for absorption). In addition, certain fatty acids, the compounds which form triglycerides by combining in groups of three, are essential nutrients—linoleic and linolenic acids, found in plant oils.

While everyone is still worried about reducing fat intake, the evidence suggests that it is the type of fat you eat, rather than the amount, which determines the impact on health. Currently, a diet that is moderate in fat, around 30 percent of total energy, and emphasizes monounsaturated fat is considered the healthy choice. Saturated fat, the type which predominates in animal products, is associated with higher blood cholesterol levels, which in turn increase the risk for heart disease. Table 1.4 shows the sample diet we used for the carbohydrate count in Table 1.3, adding in foods which add fat, and substitutions for those that usually do, in the recommended amounts.

TABLE 1.4   **Fat in a Sample Menu**

Meal	Foods	Amount	Fat (g)	Saturated Fat (g)
Breakfast	milk, 1%	1 cup	2.5	1.5
Lunch	light mayonnaise	1 tablespoon	3	1
	smoked turkey breast, fat-free	2 ounces	0	0
Dinner	sirloin tips	4 ounces	9	3.5
	olive oil	1 tablespoon	14	2
	margarine, light, in tub	1 teaspoon	2	0
Snack	milk, 1%	1 cup	2.5	1.5
	crunchy peanut butter	2 tablespoons	6	3
Total			39	12.5

Protein

This nutrient had been the darling of the diet world starting in the 1960s and continues to hold the interest of bodybuilders and other athletes. The basis for their interest is not too far-fetched: lean body mass, and specifically muscle tissue, is composed primarily of protein. While we say that protein is an essential nutrient, it is more accurate to say that the body requires specific amino acids, the building blocks of protein. Different protein-containing foods provide a mix of the various amino acids.

Protein is different from its other two energy-yielding partners, fat and carbohydrate, in that it contains the element nitrogen. A protein can contain twenty different amino acids, and when we eat protein, we get a mix of them. The body can make eleven of them on its own, but we have to eat protein containing the other nine, which are called essential amino acids.

Protein in the body is, by and large, functional. In other words, we don't have extra protein taking up space for reserve, as we do with fat. Body protein is structural, as in muscle, the inner parts of bone and hair, tendons, and other body components. But it also works, forming enzymes which pave the way for chemical reactions, immune system compounds such as antibodies, and carrier molecules (that ferry things such as vitamins in the blood). In addition to carrying nutrients in the blood, a major blood protein, albumin, is responsible for keeping the body's fluid in balance.

It's obvious, then, how important protein is. What you might not know is that the average American takes in twice as much protein as he or she needs. The recommended amount of daily protein intake is based on a person's weight. Of course, you don't add extra protein if you have excess weight. The recommended amount is 36.4 percent of body weight. A moderately active woman who weighs 120 pounds needs 43 grams of protein every day. The sample diet, at about 2,000 calories, probably works for many people and provides more than twice the amount this woman needs (see Table 1.5). This amount of excess shouldn't pose a problem for the average person, unless there is kidney disease, but you can see how calls for higher protein intakes are off base.

TABLE 1.5   **Protein in a Sample Menu**

Meal	Foods	Amount	Protein (g)
Breakfast	whole grain cereal (such as Shredded Wheat)	1 cup	5
	milk, 1%	1 cup	9
Lunch	whole wheat bread	2 slices	6
	smoked turkey breast, fat-free	2 ounces	10
Dinner	sirloin tips	4 ounces	34
	rice	1 cup	6
	stir-fry vegetables	2 cups	8
Snack	milk, 1%	1 cup	9
	crunchy peanut butter	2 tablespoons	8
	graham crackers	6	3
Total			98

Vitamins

These compounds are the stars of the nutrition world, and it was their discovery, probably more than anything else, that fueled the explosion of research into human nutrition. The current list of vitamins, thirteen to be exact, have been known to be essential for human life for several decades. However, scientists continue to study these intriguing nutrients to learn more about them—everything from how the body absorbs them from different foods to possible interactions within the body's cells. One thing is certain: as new facts unfold, new questions arise.

Although nutrition researchers still study vitamins to learn about what they do, we know some of their general roles. Some act like hormones in the body, sort of chemical messengers. Others are a part of enzymes, vital compounds that control metabolic reactions in the body. Many of the enzymes vitamins team up with can't function unless they combine with specific vitamins, called coenzymes.

A useful way to sort vitamins is into two groups: those that dissolve in fat (fat soluble) and those that dissolve in water (water soluble). This gives you some idea of how the vitamins function and how they're handled by the body. In addition, solubility determines if a vitamin can be stored in the body and how easily it's lost from the body as well as from foods during processing or preparation. And finally, knowing whether a vitamin dissolves in fat or water can give you a rough idea of which foods contain it.

You don't need much of any of the vitamins—it works out to about an ounce if you add up all the vitamins you need for a day. But scientists use different units of measure for vitamins, including mg and micrograms. Just to get an idea of how little a microgram is, one of these tiny units is equivalent to one-millionth of a gram, and a gram is about one-thirtieth of an ounce! Retinol equivalents (RE), and sometimes International Units (IU), are the measurements used in industry for vitamins A and E.

Since there are thirteen essential vitamins (fourteen, if you count the newcomer choline), our sample meal would get a bit complicated, so we'll look at two key vitamins that many Americans don't get enough of: vitamins A and C. What you'll notice is that with few exceptions, most of the significant sources of both vitamins are fruits and vegetables. One important distinction is that even in these foods, there is a wide variability in the amounts—notice that a banana and an apple provide negligible amounts of either nutrient. But the sample meal in Table 1.6 is perfectly balanced and provides our reference female with almost four times the recommended amount of vitamin A and more than seven times the vitamin C.

Minerals

Minerals are the most enduring of nutrients; that is, long after the human body has decomposed, and actually forever, the minerals in that human body will remain unchanged. Their indestructible nature tells us that cooking heat and other forms of food processing don't lower the amounts of needed minerals in our foods. However, minerals are water soluble, so prolonged contact with water will leech them out of foods. In contrast to the complex forms of the other nutrients, minerals are the basic chemical elements familiar to us in useful things other than food, such as copper pipes and iron railings.

The minerals fall into two major categories, major and trace minerals. The difference between them is a matter of amount: the body contains major minerals in amounts greater than 5 grams and less than this amount of trace minerals. This gives you an idea of the amounts you'll need to consume as well. As an example, compare the need for 800 mg of calcium, a major mineral, to that of 12 mg for the trace mineral zinc—a major difference! Table 1.7 is a list of both groups.

The roles of the minerals are diverse, with many of these nutrients doing double and triple duty. As an example, sodium, familiar

TABLE 1.6 **Vitamins A and C in a Sample Menu**

Meal	Foods	Amount	Vit. A (RE)	Vit. C (mg)
Breakfast	whole grain cereal (such as Shredded Wheat)	1 cup	0	0
	milk, 1%	1 cup	144	2
	orange juice	1 cup	50	124
	banana	1 medium	9	10
Lunch	whole wheat bread	2 slices	0	0
	smoked turkey breast, fat-free	2 ounces	0	0
	light mayonnaise	1 tablespoon	0	0
	apple	1 medium	7	8
	baby carrots, raw	2 ounces	2,024	7
Dinner	vegetable stir-fry (red pepper, onion, broccoli)	2 cups	580	296
	sirloin tips	4 ounces	0	0
	rice	1 cup	0	0
	olive oil	1 tablespoon	0	0
	margarine, light, in tub	1 teaspoon	0	0
	romaine lettuce and tomato salad	1 cup	146	14
Snack	graham crackers	6	0	0
	crunchy peanut butter	2 tablespoons	0	0
	milk, 1%	1 cup	144	2
Total			3,104	463

as the partner to chloride in table salt, helps to maintain the proper amount of acid in the blood and fluid balance outside the cells. In addition, sodium is involved in muscle contraction and nerve transmission, both vital functions considering that the heart is a muscle and has to keep beating.

As mentioned, the amount we need of each essential mineral varies depending on whether it is a major or trace mineral. Some minerals continue to prove challenging for some Americans to

TABLE 1.7 **Major and Trace Minerals**

Major Minerals	Trace Minerals
Calcium	Chromium
Chloride	Copper
Magnesium	Fluoride
Phosphorus	Iodine
Potassium	Iron
Sodium	Manganese
Sulfur	Molybdenum
Selenium	
Zinc	

consume in the recommended amounts. As for toxicity, many minerals can prove fatal in excess amounts. A deadly example is copper, which because of its potential toxicity, was the drug of choice years ago for people in India wishing to commit suicide. One reason for easy toxicity has to do with the body's handling of a particular mineral. Some minerals readily excrete into the urine when excess amounts arise, while others, such as iron, tend to accumulate in the liver, posing a considerable health risk.

If we go back to our sample day's intake and consider two minerals which pose problems for many American women, calcium and iron, we'll see that only certain types of foods provide significant amounts of each. And our sample menu again stands up to the test, providing our reference woman with about 20 percent more than the recommended amounts for calcium and iron (see Table 1.8). A final note that isn't apparent just by looking at the numbers: for several minerals, and especially for calcium and iron, the body appears to better absorb and use those nutrients from animal sources compared with grains and vegetables.

Water

Although water is so essential to life that even a few days without it can kill a person, most people don't give much thought to this vital

TABLE 1.8   **Calcium and Iron in a Sample Menu**

Meal	Foods	Amount	Calcium (mg)	Iron (mg)
Breakfast	whole grain cereal (such as Shredded Wheat)	1 cup	16	1.8
	milk, 1%	1 cup	300	1.2
	orange juice	1 cup	27	0.5
	banana	1 medium	7	0.35
Lunch	whole wheat bread	2 slices	40	1.9
	smoked turkey breast, fat-free	2 ounces	0	0.7
	light mayonnaise	1 tablespoon	0	0
	apple	1 medium	10	0.25
	baby carrots, raw	2 ounces	19	0.36
Dinner	vegetable stir-fry (red pepper, onion, broccoli)	2 cups	145	1.9
	sirloin tips	4 ounces	12	3.81
	rice	1 cup	20	2.48
	olive oil	1 tablespoon	0	0
	margarine, light, in tub	1 teaspoon	0	0
	romaine lettuce and tomato salad	1 cup	20	0.62
Snack	graham crackers	6	9	1.54
	crunchy peanut butter	2 tablespoons	11	0.54
	milk, 1%	1 cup	300	1.2
Total			936	19.15

nutrient. And while everyone knows the importance of vitamins and minerals, people may not realize that water, along with those nutrients and fat, carbohydrate, and protein, together make up the six nutrients essential for human life.

Water is a very simple compound from a chemical standpoint, consisting of only two atoms of hydrogen and one of oxygen. However, its simplicity gives rise to functions which support every aspect of human physiology, the most basic being a near perfect solvent and the medium for most of the body's chemical reactions. In addition, water brings nutrients to each cell and carries away the cell's waste products. It is part of the chemical structure of cells, tissues, and organs. Water also acts as a lubricant and cushion for joints and lubricates the digestive tract and other mucosal tissues. Another important role is in body temperature regulation because of its ability to change temperature slowly.

The need for water is based on caloric intake, and therefore body size. Under normal conditions, the average adult needs about one milliliter for every calorie consumed, or about 13.6 milliliters per pound of body weight. However, fluid requirements are affected by factors such as internal and external temperature, physical exertion, and environmental humidity level. In addition, several compounds and certain conditions can act as diuretics to promote fluid loss or cause retention of body fluid.

Naturally occurring diuretic compounds include caffeine, alcohol, and chemicals found in certain vegetables such as asparagus. Compounds which promote retention of water include high salt intake and the body's production of certain hormones, such as antidiuretic hormone and vasopressin. A person's age also influences the need for fluid, with infants requiring a higher proportion because their body composition includes a higher amount of water.

Many people believe that they need to drink eight glasses of water every day to maintain proper fluid balance, which is an erroneous assumption based on overlooking the fluid contained in foods. Most foods consist of 50 to 90 percent water, which provides about 60 percent of the adult need for water. Foods such as fruits and vegetables contain the most fluid, so depending on intake, fluid provided by foods can vary. Additionally, although drinking plain water can be beneficial, it is not essential, since other beverages contain water. Exceptions include coffee and other caffeine-containing beverages and alcohol, which because of their diuretic effect tend to deplete fluid beyond the amount they provide.

Our reference woman who eats the sample menu is taking in about 2,000 calories. This means her fluid need is 2,000 ml, or 66.6 ounces. Looking at the water contained in just the beverages, two cups of milk and one cup of juice, she has already consumed 21.6 ounces, since both milk and juice are about 90 percent water. If we only give her credit for her apple, banana, and carrots, now she's up to about 30 ounces, which doesn't include the additional water from other foods. Another four and a half cups of any liquid, including water, puts her where she needs to be.

Anything Else in There?

By now, you may be wondering about some of the other substances you've heard of in the news lately: fiber, phytoestrogen, flavonoids, and many more. Scientists refer to these as nonnutrients, of which the phytochemicals are one type. The word *nonnutrient* simply means that the compound is not one of the known nutrients which we need, while phytochemicals have some kind of activity in the body (see Table 1.9). There is increasing evidence that some of these compounds may be beneficial in preventing chronic diseases. But not all of these nonnutrients are helpful: cabbage and other plants contain compounds called goitrogens that interfere with the thyroid hormone, possibly causing a goiter. Fortunately, the heat from cooking destroys these compounds, so it's not normally a problem. Scientists who study toxins (toxicologists) tell us that plant foods are rife with potentially toxic substances.

Most of the consumer excitement regarding phytochemicals may seem recent, but food scientists have known for some time of their existence. Other nonnutrients have been acknowledged for several decades, such as dietary fiber. Although evidence continues to mount that different types of fiber are beneficial for human health, from aiding normal bowel function to preventing colon cancer, strictly speaking, fiber is not an essential nutrient. In other words, humans could theoretically survive without it. Quality of life, however, might be another matter!

The consideration of nonnutrients seems to pose another question: How do nutrition scientists figure out if something is an essential nutrient? Part of the answer relates to the history of vitamin discovery, which we'll save for upcoming chapters. But more recently, scientists have used a combination of the various types of studies to determine essentiality. Animal studies are the most obvious choice because of the method researchers use. To find out if a nutrient is essential, they feed the animal a diet, usually a formula, devoid of that compound but containing all the other nutrients they know to be essential. If the animal can grow, develop normally, and not suffer any ill effects, the compound is not essential. If the animal shows signs of deficiency, the compound is an essential nutrient.

Human case studies have also proved invaluable, usually the result of trial and error. In the not too distant past, say, forty years ago, scientists developed methods of feeding people who couldn't eat normally. Eating normally means taking food through the mouth and all the way through the intestinal tract. Doctors had to figure out another route for feeding people who had a problem somewhere in the intestinal tract. Over the years, they've refined the methods by feeding people either through a tube inserted somewhere into the intestinal tract or, for people with a nonfunctioning intestine, directly into the bloodstream. You can see, then, that they learned fairly early on what nutrients had to be added to the formulas to prevent nutrient deficiencies. Although technology has advanced greatly, some questions remain about other compounds the formulas still might need.

How Does Your Diet Add Up?

To get the most out of this book, you may want to consider doing a bit of detective work about your diet. Completing the following form will enable you to do the "How Your Diet Adds Up" quiz at the end of each section relating to a specific vitamin. The first rule

TABLE 1.9   **Well-known Nonnutrients and Phytochemicals**

	Where Is It?	*Claim to Fame*
Allyl Sulfides	chives, garlic, onions	prevent cancer and heart disease
Bioflavonoids	fruits, spices, tea, vegetables	prevent cancer and heart disease
Capsaicin	hot pepper	prevents cancer
Conjugated linoleic acid*	hamburger, butter, cheese	prevents cancer and heart disease, prevents obesity
Dithiolthiones, Indoles, Sulforaphane	broccoli, brussels sprouts, cabbage, cauliflower, kale, mustard greens	prevent cancer and heart disease
Isoflavones, Genistein, Phytosterols	soy protein	prevent tumor growth, lower blood cholesterol, replace estrogen
Lignans	soy products, flax, linseed	prevent tumor growth, lower blood cholesterol, replace estrogen
Lutein	spinach, kale, collard greens	prevents cancer
Lycopene	tomatoes, watermelon, pink grapefruit	prevents prostate cancer
Phenols	green tea, red wine	antioxidant: prevent cancer and heart disease
Phytic Acid	legumes, soy, whole grains, plant seeds	antioxidant: prevents cancer
Reversitrol	grapes	lowers blood cholesterol
Saponins	soy, legumes	antioxidant: prevent cancer and heart disease

*Actually a kind of linoleic acid (which is a nutrient), but in a different chemical form.

of thumb for keeping a food record is to do as many days as possible. It's best to do a minimum of three, and consider two weekdays and one weekend day. The more days you evaluate, the more likely your intake for that time is representative of your diet in general. The reason for including a weekend day is that most people eat differently then. Try to avoid using a day that is not typical for you, such as a special occasion (a wedding or a party).

The second rule is to make sure you write in the foods as soon as possible after eating, because most of us can barely remember what we had for dinner yesterday! And finally, try using measuring cups and spoons. You'd be surprised how much dressing you actually poured on last night's salad (see Fig. 1.2).

Here's how to do it:

1. Decide which days to include; try to keep the record for at least three days. Remember to skip days that are truly not typical for you. Enter the date under the date column.
2. Write down each food or beverage item and the amount as soon after eating as possible. For combination items, such as tuna casserole, try to include major ingredients, listed separately. If you ate at a restaurant, you'll have to write the basic item.
3. At the end of the day, review the record to make sure you didn't forget something.
4. After you've collected the number of days you wanted, you'll use these to evaluate your diet for specific vitamins. For most, you'll take an average of the total days to come up with one representative day.

FIGURE 1.2   **Food Record Form to Evaluate Your Dietary Intake**

DAY 1

Date	Food/Beverage	Amount

FIGURE 1.2 (Continued)

DAY 2

Date	Food/Beverage	Amount

DAY 3

Date	Food/Beverage	Amount

THREE-DAY AVERAGE

Food/Beverage	Number of Servings				*(Divide 3-day total by 3)* 3-Day Average
	Day 1	Day 2	Day 3	3-Day Total	3-Day Average
Breads/Grains/Cereals					
whole grain product	_____	_____	_____	_____	_____
enriched, not whole grain	_____	_____	_____	_____	_____
serving size					
bread: 1 slice					
cereal: 1 cup or ½ cup if whole grain)					
pasta: ½ cup					

(Continued)

27

FIGURE 1.2 **(Continued)**

| Food/Beverage | Number of Servings | | | | (Divide 3-day total by 3) |
	Day 1	Day 2	Day 3	3-Day Total	3-Day Average
Fruits					
citrus (orange/grapefruit/ kiwi)	___	___	___	___	___
other	___	___	___	___	___
serving:					
1 piece fresh (medium size)					
½ cup canned or 100 percent juice					
Vegetables					
dark green/orange/red	___	___	___	___	___
other	___	___	___	___	___
serving size:					
½ cup cooked; 1 cup raw					
Protein Foods					
fish or legumes	___	___	___	___	___
other	___	___	___	___	___
serving size:					
3 ounces for lean meats					
1 cup for cooked legumes					
Dairy Foods	___	___	___	___	___
serving size:					
1 cup milk/yogurt					
1 ounce for cheeses					
Fats and Sweets	___	___	___	___	___
serving size:					
1 teaspoon for oil, margarine					
1 tablespoon for salad dressing					

Chapter **Two**

Dietary Standards and Recommendations

How Do We Know How Much?

His gaze was direct and almost a challenge as this athletic, business-suited yuppie uttered a demand before we had even sat down to our first nutrition counseling session. "Look, just tell me what I gotta eat and how much to get my cholesterol down by fifty points—fast." I had never quite mastered the inscrutable "counselor" look: my overly expressive Italian face usually reflects my emotional response, which, in this case, ran the gamut of surprise at his fierce determination to more than a bit of annoyance at his obvious disdain for the complexity of making lasting nutritional changes. But in the next few seconds, I decided that I admired his faith in both nutrition science and a dietitian's ability to deliver the goods. It also shows the public's desire for specific recommendations and guidelines on a healthy diet.

Most members of generation X are too young to remember when there were only four basic food groups. That phrase harkens back to the days when junior high students, at least girls, were taught to cook and admonished to memorize the "Basic 4." As the focus shifted from nutritional deficiency to excessive intake linked to chronic disease, however, new paradigms for recommendations became vital. The starting point for dietary recommendations, the Recommended Dietary Allowances (RDAs), have evolved, often contentiously, over the last half of this century. In fact, they are currently being updated and renamed Dietary Reference Intakes (DRIs).

The RDA have been and continue to be the best yardstick we have to evaluate dietary intake. Their objective is to suggest a level of intake for many essential nutrients that is as close to adequate as possible for as many people as possible. You can probably see the difficulty inherent in coming up with one number, say for vitamin A, that is appropriate for an entire nation! This is an unavoidable design flaw, and one that should be taken into account, but not one that should preclude confidence in and use of the RDA.

In addition to a yardstick for adequacy, we also need something that translates the latest scientific knowledge about nutrition and disease into understandable and usable guidelines. As research continued to accumulate, the government stepped up to the plate and issued the Dietary Guidelines for Americans. These seven simple recommendations have since been revised and expanded on, and have spurred other health organizations to develop their own dietary guidelines; we have recommendations from the American Heart Association, the American Cancer Society, and a few others for good measure. Contrary to some public opinion, dietary recommendations from the government and most health agencies seem to converge on similar themes.

DRIs and RDAs: How Do They Come Up with These Things?

Currently, the newly revised recommendations, DRIs, cover the following nutrients: calcium, phosphorus, fluoride, magnesium, vitamin D, and the B vitamins. The RDAs for the remaining essential nutrients will be updated in the next year or so and we still need to use the old RDA until the update is complete. So we'll talk about both DRIs and RDAs, which you can consider almost one and the same.

The RDA for vitamins and the other essential nutrients are established by a subcommittee of the Food and Nutrition Board (FNB) of the National Research Council (NRC) and the National Academy of Sciences (NAS). The current DRIs are being updated by the Institute of Medicine. The NAS is a government agency, but the DRI committee, like the RDA committee before it, is made up of independent researchers representing various specialties in the field of nutrition. That's important, not just because a lot of people don't trust the government, but because the people who generate the RDA have broad expertise and experience and bring an unbiased view to the table.

The committee reviews the current information available from animal, human, and population studies and develops recommendations for nutrient intake. A recommendation is made for each nutrient in terms of the daily amount different groups of people need; the current DRI groups, which will cover all nutrients within the next few years, include:

- pregnant and lactating women (different age groups within each)
- infants: 0 to 6 months; 6 months to a year
- children: 1 to 3 years; 4 to 8; 9 to 13
- males: 14 to 18; 19 to 30; 31 to 50; 51 to 70; over 70
- females: 14 to 18; 19 to 30; 31 to 50; 51 to 70; over 70

The RDA for a nutrient includes what's called a "margin of safety," to account for individual human variation and differences in how well the body is able to absorb the nutrient from various food sources. Most experts believe that the RDAs, which are only applicable to healthy people, probably cover up to 95 percent of the American population. A small number of people will not get enough of a particular nutrient if they take in the RDA, and others will get more than they need.

So where does that leave you? The best use of the RDA is to plan or evaluate diets for groups of people, such as in a nursing home or school. But as long as we recognize their limitations, it is reasonable to use the RDA to assess an individual's diet. In fact, dietitians do it all the time; we just need to remember that while the RDA is our best estimate, that's all it is.

Not all nutrients have an official RDA; some have other classifications. For example, the RDAs are not necessarily optimal intakes, but they aren't minimum intakes, either. In other words, they are not set at a level to simply prevent a deficiency; they include an ample margin of safety. But for sodium, chloride, and potassium, an "Estimated Minimum Requirement" is set at a level which is the minimum you need with no margin of safety. Nutrients with an RDA under the 1989 RDA or the new DRI include protein and the vitamins and minerals listed in Table 2.1.

If studies show that a nutrient is essential but the experts feel that there isn't enough information to set an RDA, they suggest a range of intake with a special name. The 1989 RDA used the term Estimated Safe and Adequate Daily Dietary Intake (ESADDI). The nutrients still covered in this category include the trace minerals

TABLE 2.1   **The Essential Nutrients with RDA or DRI**

Fat Soluble Vitamins	Water Soluble Vitamins	Minerals
vitamin A	vitamin C	calcium
vitamin D	thiamin	phosphorus
vitamin E	riboflavin	magnesium
vitamin K	niacin	iron
	vitamin B_6	zinc
	folate	iodine
	vitamin B_{12}	selenium
	biotin	
	choline*	

*Some experts classify choline as a B vitamin, although it does not share its basic attributes.

chromium, molybdenum, copper, and manganese. When the committee revises recommendations for these nutrients in the future,
more research may provide solid evidence for establishing an RDA.
The new DRI uses a similar category called Adequate Intake (AI),
and has used that term for several nutrients which received
updated recommendations.

The first RDAs were published in 1943, and the plan was to
revise them every five years. In 1985, the RDAs were scheduled for
revision, but because of scientific controversy, the update didn't
appear until 1989. The word *controversy* doesn't do justice to the
brouhaha which stormed across universities and research centers
around the country, resulting in several lawsuits! The new DRIs
evolved from years of proposals and revisions for updating the
RDAs and differ in two important ways. The first change is that the
DRIs represent one combined set of North American recommendations. Previously, Canadians had their own guidelines, similar to
our RDAs. The second important change is that where the previous RDAs were designed to prevent deficiency, the new recommendations reflect current knowledge of nutrient amounts
needed to promote optimal health and prevent chronic disease.
The plan calls for revision of all nutrient recommendations in a
seven-step process, by groups of nutrients. As mentioned, new
numbers were recently issued for nutrients involved in bone
health—calcium, magnesium, phosphorus, vitamin D, and fluoride, as well as the B vitamins.

The DRIs include different categories, just as the RDAs, to
account for the more tenuous nature of the research for certain
nutrients. In addition, they will continue to include the margin of
safety, but with the DRI showing that value in the new AI category. The AI consists of the average intake that covers half the
needs of those within a specific gender and age group. Another
new category will address the increasing use of nutrient supplements and food fortification, by indicating the upper level of
safety for some nutrients.

DRI Categories

Estimated Average Requirement (EAR)

Intake that meets the needs of half the individuals in a specific group. This figure is used to develop new RDAs for some nutrients.

Recommended Dietary Allowance (RDA)

These values are derived from EARs. The RDAs are the EAR with an added amount that accounts for the variation in nutrient needs within life-stage groups (margin of safety). The RDAs will meet the need for almost all healthy individuals within a life-stage group.

Adequate Intakes (AI)

For many nutrients, the research data are not available to estimate an average nutrient requirement. For these nutrients, the DRIs give an AI recommendation which appears adequate to sustain a desired indicator for health.

Tolerable Upper Intake Level (UL)

Widespread use of supplements and food fortification has prompted the NAS to include a value that represents the best estimates of maximum intakes that do not pose risks of adverse health effects in healthy individuals within a life-stage group.

One final note about the DRIs/RDAs is that, in addition to specific nutrients, there is an RDA for daily energy or caloric intake. Because of the problem of obesity in this country, the energy RDA does not include a margin of safety. Instead, the RDAs are set at average levels for each age and gender group plus or minus 20 percent to account for either situations of higher need, as with increased physical activity, or periods of lower needs, such as occur in aging. What this means for you is that if you're average for your age and gender, in body size and activity level, the energy RDA is probably close to your actual energy needs. The reference woman at age 19 to 24 is 5'5" and weighs 128 pounds, while the reference man is 5'10", weighing 160 pounds.

The Dietary Guidelines: Can We All Agree?

The Dietary Guidelines first appeared on the scene back in 1980. The purpose was to help Americans make food choices that would prevent poor diets which research began linking to chronic diseases. These nutrition recommendations were a joint effort of two government agencies, the U.S. Departments of Agriculture and Health and Human Services (USDA, USDHHS). Since their inception, they've been both applauded and panned, but the guidelines have endured to be revised most recently in 1995.

The latest guidelines appear to be a bit more relaxed, cutting Americans some slack on previously frowned-on food ingredients such as sugar and salt. This left some nutrition advocates jeering. But in the words of one USDHHS official, the new Dietary Guidelines promote "moderation over marathons" and suggest that Americans consider *realistically attainable* health and dietary goals.

The U.S. Dietary Guidelines for Americans

- Eat a variety of foods.
- Balance the food you eat with physical activity. Maintain or improve your weight.
- Choose a diet with plenty of grain products, vegetables, and fruits.
- Choose a diet low in fat, saturated fat, and cholesterol.
- Choose a diet moderate in sugars.
- Choose a diet moderate in salt and sodium.
- If you drink alcoholic beverages, do so in moderation.

The major changes in the evolution of the Dietary Guidelines involve an emphasis on the benefit of vegetarian diets, which is included in the text for the first guideline, the more realistic focus on weight maintenance rather than attainment of ideal weight, and a more positive wording for the guidelines on salt and sugar. Another change came not in the wording of the guideline concerning alcohol, but in the accompanying text, which points to recent studies that tout the possible benefits of moderate alcohol consumption. Also in the text of the publication is another reference to recent research promoting the importance of folic acid for pregnant women.

The revised Dietary Guidelines evoked this less-than-positive characterization of the government's role from one nutrition advocate: "It's laissez-faire or do-nothing behavior. Guidelines should tell people what's the best possible diet and urge them to move in that direction. These don't."

Others, however, have commented more positively on specific aspects of the guidelines which emphasize the importance of physical activity in weight maintenance. The new guidelines recommend that Americans engage in thirty minutes of moderate physical activity every day, providing examples such as gardening, housework, or brisk walking. The rationale for this guideline follows the general tenor which stresses a more realistic approach rather than ideal goals.

While the new Dietary Guidelines for Americans may be too moderate for everyone, the USDHHS secretary's summarizing comments may be welcomed by consumers who've been overburdened with stringent preaching: "We Americans should eat a wide variety of foods, balance diet with physical activity, and use good judgment in our consumption of sugar, salt, and alcohol."

Food Labeling: Putting the Guidelines to Use

Pick up a package of fudge cookies and you'll get more information than you probably want to know: the label will probably tell you that if you eat two servings, you'll use up your fat allotment for the entire day! If you're like most people, you'll eat the cookies anyway, but at least you're informed. That didn't used to be the case. Prior to 1993, the food labeling laws hadn't kept pace with nutrition research.

Just as the RDAs had centered on adequacy and preventing nutrient deficiency, so too did the food label. You'd have information on riboflavin, thiamin, and a host of other nutrients that aren't the problem of the average American, but not a word on saturated fat and salt. In addition, manufacturers didn't have to include nutrition information unless they made a product claim. Under prodding from Congress, the Food and Drug Administration (FDA) came up with a new food label, Nutrition Facts. The FDA fixed most of the problems with the old labels, especially by mandating that virtually all food products had to include nutrition information. The exceptions include raw, single ingredient foods, fresh fruits, vegetables, and raw fish, which have voluntary nutrition information at the grocery store shelf.

It's worth taking a close look at Nutrition Facts, because you can use it to make decisions about the products you buy and how to integrate them into a healthy diet. The food label highlights key nutrients, especially those linked to prevention of chronic disease, including vitamins such as C and A. The nutrient amounts in your cookies show up as percentages of what you should eat in one day, called Daily Values (see Fig. 2.1).

Daily Values, in turn, consist of two sources which don't show up on the label, Reference Daily Intakes (RDIs) and Daily Reference Values (DRVs), but it's important to know what they represent. RDIs are the old U.S. RDAs which used an even older source, the 1968 RDAs. The DRVs are specific recommendations for nutrients which didn't have an RDA, highlighting those linked to disease, either positively or negatively: fat, saturated fat, salt, fiber, sugars, and others.

These are the nutrients which manufacturers must include on the label; they were selected because of current health issues:

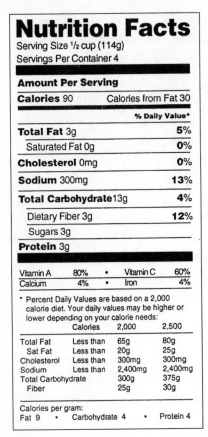

Nutrition Facts

Serving Size ½ cup (114g)
Servings Per Container 4

Amount Per Serving

| Calories 90 | Calories from Fat 30 |

	% Daily Value*
Total Fat 3g	5%
Saturated Fat 0g	0%
Cholesterol 0mg	0%
Sodium 300mg	13%
Total Carbohydrate 13g	4%
Dietary Fiber 3g	12%
Sugars 3g	
Protein 3g	

| Vitamin A | 80% | • | Vitamin C | 60% |
| Calcium | 4% | • | Iron | 4% |

* Percent Daily Values are based on a 2,000
calorie diet. Your daily values may be higher or
lower depending on your calorie needs:

	Calories	2,000	2,500
Total Fat	Less than	65g	80g
Sat Fat	Less than	20g	25g
Cholesterol	Less than	300mg	300mg
Sodium	Less than	2,400mg	2,400mg
Total Carbohydrate		300g	375g
Fiber		25g	30g

Calories per gram:
Fat 9   •   Carbohydrate 4   •   Protein 4

FIGURE 2.1

Nutrition Facts Food Label

- total calories
- calories from fat
- total fat
- saturated fat
- cholesterol
- sodium
- total carbohydrate
- dietary fiber
- sugars
- protein
- vitamin A
- vitamin C
- calcium
- iron

If a claim is made on the label about other nutrients not on the mandatory list, such as potassium or monounsaturated fat, the manufacturer must provide the information. In addition, if the product contains a nutrient either by fortification or enrichment, it must include that information.

One of the main gripes from critics is the fact that the DRVs are based on a daily intake of 2,000 calories. This is obviously a compromise, since caloric needs vary greatly from one group of the population to another. However, one of the reasons for settling on 2,000 is that increasing the energy level would increase the fat allowance, possibly encouraging higher fat intakes.

Nutrition Facts shows standardized serving sizes for various types of products for the first time. In past years, the manufacturer decided on what serving size to base the nutrient analysis. This led to what appeared to some consumers as a slightly deceptive practice, when, for example, a serving size of cereal equaled one-fourth of a cup. It was true that there were only 5 grams of fat in a serving, but most people would tend to eat four times that amount, thus acquiring a hefty 20 grams of fat at almost a third of the daily allotment.

The FDA has also restricted the use of product health claims for a list of seven nutrient/disease relationships. The claim must also be worded in such a way as to accurately reflect the relationship between the nutrient, the disease, and the nutrient's relative importance in the total diet. The approved relationships include:

- calcium and osteoporosis
- fat and cancer
- saturated fat and cholesterol and heart disease
- fiber-containing fruits, vegetables, and grain products and cancer
- fiber-containing fruits, vegetables, and grain products and heart disease
- sodium and hypertension
- fruits and vegetables and cancer

Food Guide Pyramid: A Practical Guide to Putting It All Together

The story began rather innocuously in 1988 when the USDA began development and testing of a graphic tool for use in communicating the messages of the Dietary Guidelines for Americans. But what followed seemed more like the shoot-out at the O.K. Corral than anything else. After the smoke had cleared, a pyramid loomed on the American horizon with the battle lines still drawn.

Some bystanders wondered what all the fuss was about since government agencies had been issuing dietary recommendations for years, beginning with the RDAs and culminating in the revised Dietary Guidelines for Americans. After all, the triangular figure

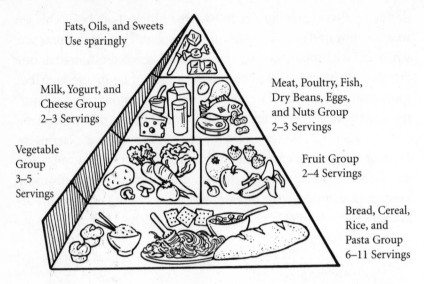

Fats, Oils, and Sweets
Use sparingly

Milk, Yogurt, and
Cheese Group
2–3 Servings

Meat, Poultry, Fish,
Dry Beans, Eggs,
and Nuts Group
2–3 Servings

Vegetable
Group
3–5
Servings

Fruit Group
2–4 Servings

Bread, Cereal,
Rice, and
Pasta Group
6–11 Servings

FIGURE 2.2   **Food Guide Pyramid: A Guide to Daily Food Choices**

with suggested serving sizes and attractive clips of foods seemed innocent enough. But it was the very shape of the image and the message it projected that sent trade industry groups to the battle-front. The intent of the pyramid was to emphasize certain food groups, such as grain products and fruits and vegetables, while deemphasizing other groups, such as meat and dairy products, and conveying a sense of what proportions the groups should represent in one's diet (see Fig. 2.2).

The USDA stated that a graphic image was needed to rein-force the messages of the Dietary Guidelines. The Dietary Guidelines call for increased consumption of complex carbohy-drates and reduced intake of fats, saturated fats, cholesterol, sugar, and salt. Because animal sources contain predominantly saturated fat and cholesterol, these foods are deemphasized in a diet based on the guidelines.

In response, industry groups marketing these foods cited the availability and promotion of newer low-fat versions of old American

staples, such as extra-lean ground round and nonfat dairy products. They pointed to the nutrient density of these products and
challenged their position on the new pyramid, which had placed
animal-derived foods directly below the fats and sweets group at
the tip of the structure. The message of the pyramid is that grain
products such as bread, cereal, and rice should form the bulk of the
diet, accounting for most of the calories provided. Next are the
fruits and vegetables, providing key vitamins and minerals. Toward
the top are the foods which should be eaten more reservedly—the
meat and dairy group. At the very top are the fats and sweets, with
the admonition "to be used sparingly."

Actually, the pyramid is not an American invention, having
first appeared in Sweden in the mid-1980s and later in Australia in
1987. Both of these countries used the figure to convey their very
similar versions of dietary guidelines. Critics had complained that
the shape of the pyramid would confuse people because the top of
something is usually the best. In the case of the "Eating Right
Pyramid," as it was later coined, in the top position were the foods
to avoid. Some educators proposed that the pyramid be inverted to
avoid this confusion. However, the USDA reported having conducted exhaustive testing and evaluation of the graphic with individuals and focus groups, much the same as marketing experts do
in the business world. They stated that there were no significant
findings related to shape inversion.

Although the pyramid has many supporters, some groups still
are not convinced that it can be effective and not misrepresent certain foods. The unveiling took longer than expected, more because
of objections from the food industry than efforts to test and polish
the pyramid. Some critics have come up with their own pyramids:
the Mediterranean Diet Pyramid, the Asian Pyramid, the Vegetarian
Pyramid, and the Oldways Pyramid, which is based on plant foods.
The USDA Center for Nutrition Policy and Promotion recently
issued informational fact sheets outlining the differences between
its pyramid and new ones on the scene in an effort to resolve

consumer confusion. It pointed to its chief advantages over its competitors—broader choices of foods and specific suggestions for number of servings from each group.

One of the long-term goals for the pyramid is widespread recognition among American consumers, and a recent survey showed that awareness increased from 58 to 67 percent of Americans within the past few years. Countless nutrition educators, those working with groups from children to the elderly, have found it to be a fun and effective teaching tool in imparting the nutrition and health recommendations of the Dietary Guidelines for Americans.

To find out if your diet stacks up to the pyramid, you need to know how many calories you should be taking in. For this, you'll need to fill in the form at the end of this section. At the end of the chapter, you'll need to review your diet record sheets (see Figure 1.2 on page 26) to evaluate your current intake compared to the recommendations in this chapter.

No one is sure how much someone should weigh to promote health, since being either too thin or too fat are both associated with health risk. But Figure 2.3 provides a rule of thumb to estimate a reasonable weight for you.

FIGURE 2.3　Determining Your Reasonable and Healthy Weight

Men:	Give yourself 106 pounds for the first 5 feet of your height, then add 6 more pounds for every inch over 5 feet. For example:
	Bob is 5'10", so a reasonable weight for him would be:
	106 pounds for his 5 feet, plus 6 pounds for each of the 10 inches
	$106 + (6 \times 10) = 166$
	You can add or subtract 10% to account for differing frame size:
	10% of 166 = ≈ 17 pounds, so the weight range for a man who is 5'10" is anywhere between 149 and 183 pounds.
Women:	Give yourself 100 pounds for the first five feet of your height, then add to the 100 pounds, 5 more pounds for every inch over 5 feet. For example:
	Carol is 5'4", so a reasonable weight for her would be:

FIGURE 2.3 (Continued)

100 pounds for her 5 feet plus 5 pounds for each of the 4 inches

$100 + (5 \times 4) = 120$

To account for differing frame size, establish the 10% range:

10% of 120 = 12 pounds, so the weight range for a woman who is 5'4" is anywhere between 108 and 132 pounds.

Step 1: Determining a Reasonable Weight

Height _____   Reasonable weight (based on formula):

Weight _____   _____

Age _____   10% add/subtract for range:

Gender _____   _____

Step 2: Determining Your Activity Level

Energy Needs: You need to estimate your level of activity, since the amount of physical activity you do each day helps to determine the energy you need, which is measured in calories.

Activity Level	Description	Calories Used Per Pound
very active	light housework, yardwork plus 30 to 60 minutes of aerobic exercise every day	17
moderately active	light housework, yardwork plus 30 to 60 minutes of aerobic exercise 3 to 4 times/week	15
inactive	some walking each day, but sitting most of the time and no regular exercise regimen	13

Step 3: Determining Your Energy Needs (how many calories you need each day)

Multiply the reasonable weight you came up with by the calories per pound which described your activity level; for an example, let's go back to Carol. She works in an office as an accountant and exercises three times each week with an aerobics group at the local community center. That would put her at the moderately active level, so we would use 15 calories for every pound of her weight of 120:

15 calories/pound × 120 pounds = 1,800 calories

Our formula gives us 1,800 calories per day, which is close to where the Pyramid puts Carol with these categories to estimate calorie intake. The Pyramid gives three ranges of caloric intake so you can determine the number of servings from each group that are right for you (see Table 2.2).

TABLE 2.2 **The Food Group Servings That Are Right for You**

Age/Gender Group:	Women, Some Older Adults	Children, Teen Girls, Active Women, Most Men	Teen Boys, Active Men
Calorie level: (Servings from food groups)	1,600	2,200	2,800
Bread and cereal	6	9	11
Vegetable	3	4	5
Fruit	2	3	4
Milk	3	3	3–4
Meat	5 ounces	6 ounces	7 ounces

Other Dietary Recommendations

The government isn't the only group to issue nutrition recommendations; a host of public and private agencies have thrown their hats into the ring. We'll look at diet guides from a private agency, the American Heart Association, and a joint effort, the 5-a-Day program.

American Heart Association Recommendations

The American Heart Association (AHA) recently released updated guidelines for Americans in its battle to prevent cardiovascular disease (CVD), diseases of the heart and blood vessels such as heart attack, high blood pressure, and stroke. The new guidelines build on previous recommendations, especially the Dietary Guidelines for Americans.

The AHA points out in the preamble to its guidelines that although its focus is the prevention of CVD, the recommendations are consistent with those issued for the prevention and treatment of other major killers such as some forms of cancer, kidney disease, and diabetes. The recommendations are geared toward reducing well-established risk factors for CVD, which include:

- the elimination of cigarette smoking
- appropriate levels of caloric intake and physical activity to prevent obesity and reduce weight in those who are overweight (especially abdominal or upper body fat)
- consumption of 30 percent or less of the day's total calories from fat
- consumption of 8 to 10 percent of total calories from saturated fatty acids
- consumption of up to 10 percent of total calories from polyunsaturated fatty acids
- consumption of 15 percent of total calories from monounsaturated fatty acids
- consumption of less than 300 mg per day of cholesterol
- consumption of no more than 2,400 mg per day of sodium
- consumption of 55 to 60 percent of calories as complex carbohydrates
- consumption of alcohol (those for whom alcohol is not contraindicated) should not exceed two drinks, or 1 to 2 ounces of ethanol, per day

5-a-Day

What was that old-fashioned saying about an apple a day? It may have been closer to the mark than we thought, but in this case, more is better! As nutritionists have recommended shifting away from the traditional basic food groups approach to a healthy diet, various suggestions on which foods and how much have been proposed. When the Pyramid was introduced last year, amid much opposition, along with it came the 5-a-Day program focusing on fruits and vegetables. Consumers had heard a multitude of information on the benefits of increasing their consumption of these foods, but the number seems to have gotten lost in the shuffle.

The 5-a-Day program was developed in 1988 by the California Department of Health Services. The targets included retail, media, and government agencies to spread the message about the healthfulness of eating fruits and vegetables. The program proved highly successful, with more than 1,800 retail operations, agencies, and industry groups participating. At just about the same time, evidence began to mount connecting high fruit and vegetable intake to a reduced risk for several diseases. More recently, the National Cancer Institute has borrowed the California theme and promoted the 5-a-Day program as part of a national health promotion focused on reducing the risk of cancer and heart disease.

Several key national authorities, such as the National Academy of Sciences, the U.S. Department of Health and Human Services, and the USDA, have recommended that people should eat at least five servings of fruits and vegetables daily. In fact, the Dietary Guidelines for Healthy Americans actually recommend up to nine daily servings. The basis for these recommendations is the burgeoning number of epidemiologic studies which suggest that people who eat greater amounts of fruits and vegetables, in particular those which are high in the antioxidant nutrients vitamin C and beta-carotene, have a lower risk for the two major killers in the United States, cancer and heart disease.

Other researchers have been quick to point out that there are a myriad of compounds in fruits and vegetables besides vitamin C and beta-carotene which may be wholly or partially responsible for the risk reduction. Some of these include the other carotenoids: alpha-carotene, lutein, lycopene, and beta-cryptoxanthin. Additionally, fiber has been suspected of offering protection against these diseases based on several population studies. And the compounds known as indoles and dithiolthiones, from the cruciferous vegetables, such as broccoli, cauliflower, and brussels sprouts, have piqued the interest of cancer researchers in recent years.

The results of a recent study of almost 87,000 nurses point to why scientists have had difficulty in identifying a single compound which is responsible for possible protective effects. Researchers analyzed the food intake of subjects and found that those who ate five or more servings of carrots a week were 68 percent less likely to have a stroke than those who ate one serving a month at most. Apparently spinach conferred protection as well, although not to the extent that carrots did. While both carrots and spinach are high in beta-carotene, they also contain other carotenoids and fiber. In addition, other compounds in the vegetables, as yet undiscovered, could be involved in risk reduction.

The studies to date have been somewhat conflicting, with most showing reduced cancer and heart disease risk in populations with high fruit and vegetable intake, but with others not supporting this conclusion. In addition, some scientists believe that the levels needed of the antioxidant nutrients and other protective compounds to significantly lower disease risk can only be achieved with nutrient supplements. Data from one recent study support this view. Subjects had a significant reduction in risk for heart disease only when supplementing their diet with vitamin E, with dietary intake exerting no significant effects.

Failure to pinpoint the exact protective compound is the reason for encouraging an increase in fruit and vegetable consumption with the 5-a-Day campaign. In addition, most of the studies so far which have shown reduced risk for chronic disease were based on analysis of dietary intake of fruits and vegetables. However, the recommendations seem to fall on deaf ears, with a recent survey reporting fully 77 percent of Americans falling short and only 8 percent achieving the goal. Perhaps more alarming is the low percentage of Americans who are aware of the recommendation for fruit and vegetable daily intake: 34 percent thought it was one serving, 32 percent thought two servings, and 25 percent thought three to four servings.

The National Cancer Institute and other health organizations are hoping to increase awareness of the 5-a-Day recommendation. At this point, it isn't clear why Americans haven't taken to this simple advice, but the experts will keep plugging away at this worthwhile goal.

Let's Take a Closer Look at Your Diet

Now it's time to see how your diet stacks up against all of the recommendations we've just considered. It is important to remember that even a three-day intake record is not truly representative of the foods you eat over a longer period of time; but at least it's a start. We'll use a quiz format in this chapter and upcoming ones to compare the average of your three-day intake to the various recommendations, starting with the Dietary Guidelines (see Fig. 2.4).

FIGURE 2.4   **Dietary Guidelines Quiz**

Look over your 3-Day Average Intake and give yourself points as indicated for each of the seven Dietary Guidelines. Give yourself the points indicated next to each blank space in the point column, if you followed the Dietary Guideline.

Points

Eat a variety of foods: 20   _____
If you ate at least 2 servings from each food group (4 or more
from the grain group) and had at least 1 serving in the vegetable
group of dark green/orange and 1 serving in the fruit group
of citrus

Balance the food you eat with physical activity;   15   _____
Maintain or improve your weight:
If you weigh within 10% of the weight you calculated in Figure 2.3,
and exercise at least three times each week

Choose a diet with plenty of grain products, vegetables,   15   _____
and fruits:
If you ate at least 5 servings of fruits and vegetables (combined),
and at least 4 servings of grain foods

Choose a diet low in fat, saturated fat, and cholesterol: 20   _____
If you ate fish and legumes at least once in the three days, and
only 1 serving of red meat, and used oil or margarine instead
of butter, and used low-fat dairy products

Choose a diet moderate in sugars: 5   _____
If you ate an average of one dessert each day

FIGURE 2.4   (Continued)

	Points
	Points

Choose a diet moderate in salt and sodium: 5 ____
If you ate only 2 servings or less of any of the following on any
of the three days; potato chips or other salty snacks, bacon or
luncheon meats, pickles, soy sauce

If you drink alcoholic beverages, do so in moderation: 20 ____
If you drank 2 or less alcohol-containing drinks each
day if you're a man and 1 or less if you're a woman
(one drink is 4 ounces of wine, 1 ounce of liquor,
or 12 ounces of beer)   **total points:** ____

SCORE	90–100	Awesome!
	89–80	Not bad; with a bit of work you'll be on your way.
	79–70	That's about average for Americans, but who wants to be average?
	69–60	Uh oh, try reading this chapter over!

Section **Two**

Introducing . . . the Vitamins

Dr. M.'s tone on the phone was frantic as I took his call on the run before meeting with a patient he had referred to me over a month ago, now back for a follow-up. "You have to tell Mr. V. to lay off the diet. He looks like a concentration camp victim! His cholesterol is great, but he has lost too much weight!" I panicked momentarily, envisioning a once-robust father of four reduced to an emaciated shell of a man on his way to physical disaster, all because of me. I wracked my brain trying to remember if my advice could have produced this wreck, but short of a strange reaction to vitamin E, which was unheard of, nothing seemed to fit.

As it turned out, Mr. V. was actually in great shape, his modest weight loss largely responsible for the plunge in his blood cholesterol level. I chalked up Dr. M.'s overwrought reaction, deserving of an Oscar, to the shock of seeing a once-plump face taking on a new leaner look. And as for vitamin E, by adding a low-dose daily supplement, Mr. V. further reduced his previously high risk for a heart attack. Since that episode a few years back, this special nutrient has continued to wow the public and may be single-handedly responsible for the renewed interest in vitamins. These intriguing little

51

compounds were big news in their early years, but public interest can be fickle, and, as with most trends, it subsequently waned. Oddly enough, it was the seemingly improved health of Americans which rekindled interest in vitamins—a paradox which requires further explanation.

In the first years of the twentieth century, research in human nutrition revolved around the newly discovered vitamins and their role in human deficiency. But not long after, overt malnutrition and nutrient deficiency seemed to be ancient history for most Americans. As we started living longer, partly due to an abundant food supply and improved nutrition, the mortality rate for chronic or degenerative diseases began to increase.

Chronic diseases are those which develop over a lifetime, and the two major diseases of this type are cardiovascular disease and cancer, which together account for the most deaths in this country. Cardiovascular disease (CVD) refers to any disease of the heart and blood vessels, which includes heart attack and stroke; CVD is the leading cause of death in the United States. As researchers took note of this trend in mortality rates, they shifted focus to these diseases and the role of risk factors, in particular, dietary components such as fat and fiber. But more recently, vitamins have made a comeback, displacing fat and fiber as the hot topics of research, in the study of a protective role in prevention of a variety of chronic diseases.

Some of the most promising and exciting research is in the area of specific vitamins and cardiovascular disease and cancer. This is especially true in light of the changing demographics in the United States, the aging of the population. The statistics indicate that currently, one in eight Americans is over the age of sixty-five; in the year 2010, it will change to one in seven; and by 2030, one in five. This next chapter will give you a general overview of vitamins as a group of nutrients, looking at some of the similar roles they perform and how the body handles them.

Chapter *Three*

Vitamins: An Overview

The vitamin story really began hundreds of years ago when humans first recognized that specific diseases were related to eating habits. Accounts from as early as the seventh century described one such disease, beriberi, and scurvy was documented in the late thirteenth century. Although the names of some of these deficiency diseases seem comical and the diseases are rare in our population, they caused untold suffering and deaths throughout history. As time went on, people learned that certain foods could cure these diseases. But it wasn't until the turn of this century that scientists were able to identify the chemicals in foods which produced the dramatic cures.

The word *vitamin* came about from a Polish scientist, Casimir Funk, in the early 1900s. He discovered several substances that he termed vitamine, from "vital amine." An amine is a compound that contains nitrogen. Later, researchers found that not all true vitamins could be chemically classified as amines, so they dropped the "e" and kept *vitamin*. Here's the definition they decided on for a vitamin:

> An organic compound that is needed in very small amounts for growth and maintenance of life.

Their organic nature means that vitamins contain the element carbon, and this distinguishes them from another group of essential nutrients, the minerals; carbon is oxidized when combusted, while minerals retain their elemental character even if incinerated at high temperatures. This is another reason why vitamins are generally more readily destroyed by cooking and food preparation methods than their indestructible cousins, the minerals.

With this knowledge, vitamins became recognized as one of the six essential nutrients required for human life, along with water, carbohydrates, protein, fat, and minerals. As scientists discovered new vitamins, they named the compounds alphabetically: A, B, C, D, E, and K. The gaps in the list, which turned out to be rather lengthy, were due to some substances being dropped after they turned out not to be vitamins by the accepted definition. All the confusing numbers associated with the letters, like B_1 and B_2, are the result of the discovery that what initially was believed to be one compound in fact were several, each with a specific function in the body. At the present time, fourteen vitamins are recognized as being required by humans.

What Vitamins Do for You

Relay Messages

Vitamins have specialized duties in the body, but many share similar types of functions. Some vitamins serve as chemical messengers, similar to hormones. Although the term *hormone* evokes colorful images of overpowering passions, hormones control the body's internal environment by keeping the innumerable activities of cells and organs in check. The process starts when specialized groups of cells, or organs such as the pancreas, release hormones in response to a situation in the body which needs correcting. The hormone travels in the blood away from its point of origin to the target, again a group of cells or an organ, and tells the target to do something.

The easiest example to understand is that of the hormone insulin, which the pancreas releases in response to an increase in blood sugar or glucose level, such as occurs after a meal. Insulin courses through the blood and relays the message "clear glucose from the blood." This simple message causes a variety of tissues to respond in different ways, but all with the goal of reducing blood glucose. To fat cells, whose purpose is to store excess glucose as fat, the reaction is to do just that. In contrast, other cells respond by allowing glucose to enter and perhaps be used for energy, and liver cells take up the glucose and make glycogen, a storage form of the sugar, for later use. The result is that in short order, the blood glucose level returns to normal.

For an example in the vitamin family, we turn to vitamin D, which some scientists say is more properly termed a hormone. While vitamin D has an active role in bone formation, one indirect way in which it fulfills this role is to regulate calcium levels in the blood. As with most compounds in the blood, the level of calcium must remain within a narrow range. If it doesn't stay in the right range, horrific results could ensue such as tetany, a condition marked by convulsions and muscle spasms. Vitamin D acts as a hormone by telling bone tissue to give up some calcium and release it into the blood in order to raise blood calcium levels.

Help the Helpers in the Meat Grinder of Life

Another common role for some vitamins is as part of enzymes. Enzymes are special proteins that jump-start the myriad reactions in the body, much as do jumper cables from a charged battery to a dead battery in your car. Without these important compounds, it would take considerably longer, in some cases virtually forever, to start chemical reactions vital to sustaining life. A vitamin that helps an enzyme is called a coenzyme, and unless it combines with that enzyme, the enzyme can't do its job. What is its job? The answer could encompass a college-level course in nutritional metabolism, but we'll synthesize it down to a few pages that start with a cheeseburger.

Although you may have really enjoyed the taste of the burger, the ultimate goal of eating it is to fuel your body so that it can keep doing work for you. Work requires energy, and the currency of the body's energy is a small compound you may remember from biology class called ATP (adenosine triphosphate). Your body's metabolic machinery makes ATP from the foods you eat, and the processes to do this are those of metabolism. Many processes involve breaking down larger compounds, such as the protein in the burger's meat, into smaller ones. Breaking things down is called catabolism, while making new compounds is called anabolism—the two aspects of metabolism.

After you eat a cheeseburger, your digestive system begins to dismantle it so that eventually the smallest nutrient components can be absorbed into the system. Vitamins and minerals generally are present in a form in which they can enter the blood, although they often need other molecules to carry them. However, the energy-yielding nutrients of fat, carbohydrate, and protein need to be broken down even further before they can give up their energy. Digestive enzymes start the process by doing just that: enzymes in the stomach and intestine render the energy nutrients absorbable and ready for the body to metabolize into usable energy.

The building blocks of the energy nutrients in our cheeseburger, components small enough to be absorbed, include amino acids, glycerol, glucose, and fatty acids. These building blocks enter into metabolic pathways which will break them down even further into their constituent atoms. A metabolic pathway is a cycle of chemical reactions into which compounds enter and are acted on by the cycle's enzymes, changing them into more useful forms.

You might think of the pathways as meat grinders, the old-fashioned kind with the crank handle that the butcher has to continually turn in a circle. He puts chunks of meat in (those are the nutrient building blocks), and after cranking the handle, ground meat comes out in even smaller pieces than before. Depending on what he's going to do with the meat, he can put the ground meat back in to make even smaller pieces. When he's done, our butcher can fry up the meat to eat right away (and get the energy from it!), or he can store it for later use in different forms, such as sausages in the fridge or a block of ground meat in the freezer. You might think of the B vitamins as butcher assistants who stand by and take turns at the crank.

In much the same way, glucose enters into one of the metabolic pathways and gets broken down into a smaller compound called pyruvate. This smaller compound can either continue on for further breakdown all the way to energy as ATP or be recycled back into glucose in a different pathway. All of the pathways are dependent on various B vitamins because of their role as coenzymes, or helpers to enzymes, that nudge the chemical reactions in the pathways. The very first step in getting energy from glucose, splitting it into pyruvate, requires niacin. Next, thiamin and pantothenic acid in concert with niacin, help spark the cascade of energy-producing reactions that follow. And in rapid succession or in other pathways, each B vitamin joins the symphony to allow the release of energy from the cheeseburger.

A glance at the myriad of metabolic pathways would make your head spin, and it probably takes a biochemist to appreciate the beauty of the complex reactions. But it's not the vitamins' "day jobs" that generate excitement among the average man on the street, it's the possibility that they can help prevent or treat a growing list of diseases. The upcoming chapters will review each vitamin in more detail, but Table 3.1 shows the research highlights linking specific vitamins to disease.

TABLE 3.1 Vitamin Links to Preventing Specific Diseases

Fat Soluble Vitamins

Vitamin A	protection against ulcers, epithelial tissue cancers; carotenoid precursors: heart disease, cancer
Vitamin D	protection against osteoporosis, colon cancer, diabetes, osteoarthritis
Vitamin E	protection against cancer, heart disease, cataracts, Alzheimer's disease, colon cancer

Water Soluble Vitamins

Niacin	lowers blood cholesterol
Vitamin B_6/ Pyridoxine	protection against heart disease, premenstrual syndrome, carpal tunnel syndrome
Folate	protection against heart disease, neural tube defects
Vitamin B_{12}/ Cobalamine	protection against heart disease
Vitamin C/ Ascorbic Acid	protection against cancer, heart disease, cataracts

Chapter **Four**

One Way to Look at Vitamins: Fat Soluble Versus Water Soluble

V itamins conveniently fall into two classes, fat soluble and water soluble, which describe a chemical attribute: compounds either dissolve in water or in fat, and those two solvents don't mix. When you add vinegar, which is a water-based liquid, to oil, they form separate layers. But beyond a chemical trait, this classification gives you some idea of how the vitamins function and how they're handled by the body. From a practical standpoint, solubility determines if a vitamin can be stored in the body and how easily it's lost from the body and, for that matter, from foods during processing or preparation. It also gives you a tiny clue as to the foods that might contain them.

Solubility and Vitamin Clues in Foods

Let's start with how solubility tells you where to look for vitamins. A vitamin has to be dissolved in some part of a food to be contained within it, and in the case of fat-soluble vitamins, the food has to contain at least a moderate amount of fat to be a good source of one of these vitamins. One exception to this rule of thumb is a food that has been fortified with a fat soluble vitamin, such as skim milk which contains no fat. Milk naturally contains a fair amount of fat, 8 grams in one cup to be exact, and a significant amount of vitamin A. When manufacturers remove the fat, they put back in the lost vitamin A and also throw in some vitamin D. Other examples include commercial products like breakfast cereals. These cereals are made from various grains which don't naturally contain fat soluble vitamins such as vitamins A and D.

Another exception to our rule is when a food contains a precursor of fat soluble vitamin A, such as beta-carotene and other carotenoids. A precursor, sometimes called a provitamin, is a compound that the body can convert into an active vitamin. The most significant food sources of vitamin A precursors are highly colored fruits and vegetables, which tend to be very low in fat. You can eat lots of fruits and vegetables for practically no dent in your daily fat budget and get loads of carotenoids, which your body can turn into active vitamin A as you need it.

Knowing the solubility of vitamins also tells you about how easily these nutrients may be lost in food preparation, most of which occurs with the addition of water and when heating foods. In general, fat soluble vitamins are fairly well retained during food preparation, largely because they don't dissolve in water. In contrast, water soluble vitamins readily dissolve into the water used in cooking. This is one reason why the Southern practice of using pot liquor, liquid remaining after cooking foods like vegetables, to make soups and stews is a smart idea; the water soluble vitamins that escaped into the water during cooking are recycled back into something you can eat instead of being poured down the drain. Heat is a problem for many water soluble vitamins, more so for some than others. Vitamin C, folate, and riboflavin are among the touchiest vitamins. The following are tips to cut down on nutrient losses from foods during food preparation.

Food Preparation and Storage

- Use fresh produce as soon as possible after purchase, as naturally contained enzymes destroy nutrients as the produce continues to ripen.
- Avoid soaking produce in water for long periods of time.
- Leave skins intact on produce when possible (if you must peel, use a peeler to remove the least amount of flesh, since nutrients are often concentrated between the skin and flesh).
- Cut produce after washing if possible; cut into larger pieces rather than small pieces because more juice (high in water soluble vitamins) is lost with more cutting.
- Return milk in opaque plastic jugs to the fridge as soon as possible since riboflavin is readily destroyed by exposure to light; for the same reason, don't store pasta and other grains in glass containers (glass is okay if stored in the cupboard).
- Keep juices tightly covered both in fridge and out because vitamin C evaporates into the air.

Cooking

- Steam vegetables rather than boil in large quantities of water; microwaving and stir-frying are also better than boiling.
- Add vegetables to boiling water, rather than placing in water and then bringing to a boil; quickly reduce heat to a simmer.
- Limit cooking time and avoid high temperatures for all foods.
- Never rinse boiled grain products such as pasta because vitamins will also be rinsed off; to avoid stickiness, add just a touch of olive oil.

The Solubility Factor Inside the Body

In general, water soluble vitamins are not stored in the body's tissues to any great extent, so you need them every day. These vitamins are also readily excreted by the kidneys, which means that when you consume more than you need, the excess ends up in the urine. While this seems wasteful, especially if the excess amount came from supplements for which you probably paid an average of 10 to 50 cents for each tablet, you can be somewhat assured that you won't accumulate toxic amounts. In contrast, the body can store fat soluble vitamins for long periods of time and not excrete them in case of an excess. People don't often realize that too much of a good thing, even vitamins, can actually kill you!

A favorite story that college nutrition professors regale students with when they get to the vitamins lecture is the one about the Arctic explorers and polar bear livers. It seems that some of the first explorers to those cold wastelands ran out of food supplies and were forced to rely on what they could find around them for sustenance. The only edible food was an abundance of polar bear livers, which are even higher in vitamin A than other types of liver. Because they ate so much, and vitamin A is not excreted, some of them died from vitamin A toxicity—quite a vivid illustration, albeit unlikely to occur in the average town, of the potential toxicity of vitamins. Similarly, vitamin D has a fairly low toxicity range. But those are fat soluble vitamins, which one would expect to possibly cause problems.

Conventional wisdom had suggested that, in sharp contrast, water soluble vitamins were harmless in excessive amounts, as the body was able and willing to dump the overage into the daily urine for excretion. But recent studies and clinical experience have shown that excess amounts of some of the water soluble vitamins can have undesirable effects. A common example is niacin, which is modestly effective in lowering blood cholesterol. The amount needed to lower cholesterol greatly exceeds the RDA, and the nutrient megadose of up to 100 times the RDA acts like a drug in the body. The megadose produces what are called pharmacological or drug effects, and besides lowering cholesterol, it may also cause liver damage and stomach ulcers. While the water soluble vitamins are not quite as lethal as some of the fat soluble ones, excesses can cause physiologic problems. We'll explore the potential problems of each vitamin in the upcoming chapters.

An overview of vitamins would be remiss if we neglected to mention the impostors which crafty marketers slip into everything from shampoo to "high-energy snack bars." If scientists did discover a new vitamin, you'd hear about it on the 6:00 P.M. news before the story made it into print. But some of these fake vitamins sound like the real thing, like vitamin B_{15}, one of the "newly discovered" vitamins. Following is a brief list of some perennial impostors:

- Bioflavonoids, vitamin P
- Gerovital H-3
- Hesperidin
- Inositol
- Laetrile, vitamin B_{17}
- Lecithin
- Nucleic acids
- Pangamic acid, vitamin B_{15}
- Provitamin B_5 complex

Do Americans Get Enough Vitamins?

The government routinely surveys and assesses the American population for a variety of health and nutrition parameters. Surveys of food habits are extremely valuable because they give scientists an idea of the kinds and amounts of foods that the average American eats. From this information, researchers can figure out the nutrient level and the public's nutritional status, especially when they combine the dietary data with blood tests and other health information. Some of the surveys also obtain information on nutrition knowledge and behaviors. The final benefit is when health care workers such as dietitians and physicians use survey results to help identify people who might be at risk for nutritional deficiencies and to plan nutrition education programs based on the needs of most Americans.

Among the big surveys is the National Health and Nutrition Examination Survey (NHANES); several have already been completed over the past few decades. One aspect of our health that NHANES checks is our nutrient intake; they do this by asking people what they usually eat and what they've recently eaten. Then, some "lucky" researcher gets to pore over the mounds of information collected and computer-analyze the foods for nutrient content. NHANES also measures and weighs people of all ages and takes blood and urine samples to see how healthy we are.

Another government survey of the American diet is the Continuing Survey of Food Intakes by Individuals (CSFII). The most recent CSFII, known as *What We Eat in America,* covered a three-year period from 1994 to 1996 and surveyed Americans on their food consumption. In 1989, CSFII added a telephone follow-up survey to measure what Joe Consumer knows and his attitude about a healthy diet, because this influences his food choices and his nutrient intake. The recent CSFII reached 16,000 Americans and the follow-up survey, 5,000.

So what's the diagnosis? The results are mixed; most Americans seem to be getting enough of many of the essential nutrients, but some of us are falling short (see Table 4.1). Some key nutrients are nowhere near what is needed to protect against chronic diseases such as heart disease. Two vitamins which came up short are vitamin E and B_6. Also, although nutritionists have been promoting the benefits of dark green and deep yellow veggies, Americans are eating less than an ounce of these each day. On the plus side, intake of the other twelve vitamins appears to be adequate for most of us.

Although some Americans appear to be knowledgeable regarding the importance of a healthy diet and exercise, a significant number do not seem to value these contributors to health. When people were surveyed about the personal importance of each Dietary Guideline, some of the numbers were surprising in light of the experts' definition of a healthy diet: only 30 percent of men and 37 percent of women said that choosing a diet with "plenty of breads, cereals, rice, and pasta" was very important; 61 percent of men and 73 percent of women stated that choosing a diet with "plenty of fruits and vegetables" was very important. In summary, we still have a long way to go to improve our nutritional health, especially in translating what we learn into action and good habits over a lifetime. Table 4.1 shows some highlights of the CSFII.

To Supplement or Not to Supplement?

That really is the question that consumers are asking themselves these days. The old party line of most dietitians and physicians

TABLE 4.1   **Continuing Survey of Food Intakes by Individuals (CSFII) 1994–1996: "What We Eat in America"**

Average Intakes of:	Men	Women	Recommended Level
Calorie	2,500	1,600	varies by age/height
Sodium	4,000 mg*	3,000 mg*	2,400 mg
Fiber	19g	14g	20–30g

Percentage of Population Meeting 100% of RDA for Vitamins and Minerals and Recommended Level of Other Nutrients:

	Men (%)	Women (%)
Calcium	45**	21**
Magnesium	37	22
Zinc	35	17
Total fat (30% or less)	29	35
Saturated fat (10% or less)	34	41
Cholesterol (300 mg or less)	56	78

Mean Intake of Selected Vitamins for Adults as a Percentage of the RDA:

	Men (%)	Women (%)
Vitamin E	102	88
Vitamin B_6	112	72

*Does not include salt added at table, so actual amount is significantly higher.
**This data was published before the new recommendations (DRI) for calcium were developed; actual percentage of population below recommended level is higher.

went something like this: you don't need vitamin supplements—you can get everything you need from food. That stock answer doesn't work anymore because the issue has become increasingly complex. A more enlightened response would start with "that depends." Based on what the body of vitamin research tells us, supplement use can be both helpful and harmful, bringing risks as well as benefits. For some people, supplements provide more benefits than risks, so the answer will be different for each person. Let's take a look at just exactly on what the answer depends.

The starting point is the quality of your diet. Most nutrition experts would make the case, and rightly so, that a person should first seek to improve his or her diet before taking supplements. A more compelling reason for optimizing the diet is one that puts supplements in perspective. Food contains thousands of naturally occurring chemicals, some of which are essential nutrients such as vitamins, but many more of which are what scientists call phytochemicals. These compounds are proving to be disease fighters, at least in the laboratory, and evidence is growing that they may protect against disease in the real world as well. Many cannot be duplicated in the lab, and, even more important, it is likely that food contains some phytochemicals that researchers haven't yet identified. The moral of the phytochemical story is that everyone should examine his or her dietary intake and make changes that lead to a healthier diet.

However, people who don't consume many calories (for a variety of reasons) are probably missing out on nutrients. These people include perennial calorie counters or dieters as well as individuals who have chronic conditions that affect their food intake (even if only periodically). The most serious conditions are those which affect nutrient absorption such as Crohn's disease, which attacks the small intestine where nutrient absorption takes place. Any disease which causes diarrhea will result in the effective excretion of nutrients before they have a chance to be absorbed. These conditions collectively produce malabsorption and are good reasons for considering vitamin and other nutrient supplementation.

The elderly are another group of people who benefit from supplements. Many elderly people don't take in enough calories, and others may have normal aging problems such as poor dentition which cause them to limit their intake. Good evidence for the benefit of supplements for the elderly are clinical trials which used a variety of vitamins and minerals. Back in the 1980s, immunity researchers first showed that a daily multivitamin supplement prevented the occurrence of infection in the elderly. A recent French study supported the use of a vitamin and mineral supplement in the elderly, demonstrating a lower rate of infections in those taking a supplement. Although research of the elderly population and supplements to reduce infection is fairly well documented, an interesting study on colon cancer indicates that a general multivitamin supplement and extra vitamin E may help younger people avoid this disease. The study reported that men and women who used multivitamins for ten years had a 50 percent lower risk for colon cancer compared to those who didn't use a supplement. In addition, people who used at least 200 IU of vitamin E enjoyed a 57 percent lower risk compared to those who didn't take extra vitamin E.

The best direct evidence is linked to vitamin E; a study of vitamin E supplementation showed that this nutrient boosted the immune system in a group of elderly subjects. In addition, even more studies have reported that the elderly have special nutritional requirements, with higher demand for some vitamins at a time when energy needs decline. That means that the average elderly person would have to eat an even more nutritious diet than when he or she was younger to meet nutritional needs.

And finally, like Mr. V. at the beginning of this chapter, many Americans are at high risk for early death from heart disease and cancer. Many legitimate nutrition experts are now recommending that, along with a healthy diet, supplements may help push the delicate balance of health and disease in their favor. The clear monarch from the vitamin kingdom in this regard is vitamin E, which numerous studies have singled out as an aid in the prevention and even treatment of heart disease. Newer on the scene are the B vitamins, folate, B_{12}, and B_6, which can lower the blood level of homocysteine, a compound researchers have linked to heart disease risk.

A few years back, the federal government passed legislation in an effort to help consumers make informed choices about dietary supplements. The Dietary Supplement Health and Education Act of 1994 charged the Food and Drug Administration (FDA) to issue proposals for labeling of dietary supplements. Prior to this law, manufacturers of vitamin and other supplements had weaker labeling standards than dinosaur-shaped fruit snacks! After much debate from all, supplement makers, advocacy groups, and health professionals, the FDA issued these regulations:

- Labels may carry health claims only for approved nutrients and diseases. The FDA is in charge of deciding which claims are valid. Currently two claims are approved: folate helps to reduce risk for neural tube defects (birth defects such as spina bifida); calcium may reduce osteoporosis risk.
- Products can't make claims to "diagnose, treat, cure, or relieve a specific disease."
- Labels may describe nutrient functions in the body and explain how it works, and link the nutrient (if essential) to "general well-being."
- Supplement labels will be entitled "Supplement Facts" to distinguish them from food labels which are called "Nutrition Facts." This alerts consumers to the fact that labeling guidelines are different for supplements.
- A supplement will be labeled "dietary supplement" as part of its statement of identity.
- The term *high potency* may be used in reference to a particular nutrient if the supplement contains 100 percent or more of that nutrient's Reference Daily Intake (RDI) or Daily Reference Value (DRV).

- The term *antioxidants* refers to vitamins C, E, and beta-carotene when the nutrient claim consists of "good source of antioxidants."
- To be labeled as "high in antioxidants," a product must contain 20 percent or more of the RDI per serving for the aforementioned nutrients.

Is Nature a Better Chemist?

With the current buzz surrounding holistic health and all things natural, people often ask if vitamin supplements from natural sources are better than synthetic ones, which just means made in a laboratory. Vitamins are chemical compounds; the body doesn't discriminate between those that are synthesized in a laboratory and those from food sources. By the same reasoning, vitamins labeled "natural" are indistinguishable to the body from synthetic vitamins, especially in light of the fact that the term *natural* carries no legal definition.

There are, of course, a few exceptions to date—vitamin E and folate. Vitamin E exists in nature as two groups, the tocopherols and tocotrienols, and together they include at least eight additional compounds called isomers or vitamers. The tocopherols have the most vitamin activity, and of these, alpha-tocopherol is the most potent. The natural form of alpha-tocopherol is known as *RRR*-alpha-tocopherol, and the synthetic is all-rac-alpha-tocopherol. In the body, RRR-alpha has a higher activity compared to the synthetic all-rac-alpha. However, even this may be a nonissue, since the amount in supplements can compensate for this difference. Additionally, one recent study showed that both forms were equal in their antioxidant ability to fight free radicals.

The other exception, folate, prompted the Institute of Medicine to issue strong language regarding the use of supplements. The Institute of Medicine is currently in charge of revising current nutrient recommendations for Americans.

In general, then, consumers can save themselves quite a bit of money at the checkout counter, since most naturally derived vitamin supplements cost up to double that of their synthetic counterparts. Quality control may also be tighter for synthetics and the supplement more likely to be uniform and less likely to contain contaminants than one from a natural source.

Table 4.2 summarizes the role of each vitamin and symptoms of both deficiency and toxicity. Upcoming chapters will give you more detailed information on all the vitamins.

Antioxidant Nutrients Fight the Bad Boys of Disease: The War Against Free Radicals

All the vitamins play unique roles in the body, but one special ability of some vitamins is taking the spotlight—antioxidant activity. It's this activity that scientists think is the protection against a host of diseases including heart disease, cancer, and Alzheimer's disease because compounds called free radicals may be at the root of these. The next sections provide a simplified overview of how researchers think antioxidant nutrients fight disease. Three nutrients, the carotenoids, vitamin E, and vitamin C, make up the antioxidants. To understand antioxidants and how they fight disease, we need to look at the most basic level in the body, the cell.

The cell membrane is composed primarily of proteins and lipids. These lipids are polyunsaturated, a chemical term that distinguishes them from either saturated or monounsaturated fats (similar to the different forms of dietary fat that we eat). Saturation refers to hydrogen atoms, but you probably recognize these different fats as either artery friendly or the kind that raise your blood cholesterol. The polyunsaturated lipids are more susceptible to oxidation, or combining with oxygen, which generates free radicals. Free radicals are unstable compounds that keep damaging other compounds in a cascade reaction that doesn't stop until an antioxidant comes along.

TABLE 4.2   **Vitamins: Their Functions and Signs of Deficiency and Toxicity**

Chief Functions in the Body	Deficiency Symptoms	Toxicity Symptoms
Fat Soluble Vitamins		
Vitamin A		
maintains health of the cornea for vision, other epithelial cells and mucous membranes, skin and bone and teeth growth; regulates and helps synthesize hormones for reproduction; immune and cancer protection	anemia breakdown of cornea blindness diarrhea painful joints tooth decay kidney stones night blindness susceptibility to infections	anorexia (loss of appetite) bone pain growth retardation fatigue lack of bone growth headaches rashes hair loss nosebleeds blurred vision loss of menstrual cycle in females
Vitamin D		
Maintains bone tissue by regulating the absorption and excretion of calcium and phosphorus	defective bone growth bowed legs joint pain muscle spasms	headaches excessive thirst high calcium level in blood kidney stones weakness, nausea loss of appetite

TABLE 4.2 (Continued)

Chief Functions in the Body	Deficiency Symptoms	Toxicity Symptoms
Vitamin E		
Maintains cell membranes; acts as an antioxidant in fighting disease-causing free radicals and in protecting other important compounds from oxidation	anemia breast cysts leg cramps, weakness	enhances effect of anticoagulant drugs gastrointestinal and abdominal discomfort
Vitamin K		
Helps synthesize compounds involved in blood clotting and regulation of calcium levels in blood	excessive bleeding	jaundice interference of anticoagulant drugs
Water Soluble Vitamins		
Vitamin B₁		
Thiamin		
Helps the body process energy from food as part of a coenzyme; helps maintain normal appetite and function of nervous system	abnormal heartbeat enlargement of heart eventual heart failure fluid retention mental confusion paralysis wasting of muscle; pain and weakness in muscles	none documented

	Function		
Vitamin B$_2$ *Riboflavin*	Helps the body process energy from food as part of a coenzyme; helps maintain vision and skin	abnormal cornea cracking at corners of mouth sensitivity to light skin rash tongue abnormalities	none documented
Niacin *Vitamin B$_3$, Nicotinamide*	Helps the body process energy from food as part of a coenzyme; helps maintain skin, nervous, and digestive systems	anorexia diarrhea tongue abnormalities low blood pressure sweating, flushing mental confusion	diarrhea dizziness liver dysfunction skin rash weakness
Vitamin B$_6$ *Pyridoxine*	Helps the body process protein and fat from food as part of a coenzyme; helps to make red blood cells and convert an amino acid into niacin	anemia kidney stones rash, dermatitis spastic muscles, convulsions tongue abnormalities	fluid retention depression, memory loss fatigue weakness peripheral neuropathy

(Continued)

TABLE 4.2 (Continued)

Chief Functions in the Body	Deficiency Symptoms	Toxicity Symptoms
Folate Helps to make new cells as part of a coenzyme	anemia depression, mental confusion diarrhea, constipation susceptibility to infections tongue abnormalities	can mask a B_{12} deficiency
Vitamin B_{12} *Cobalamine* Helps make new cells and maintain nervous system	anemia fatigue paralysis skin abnormalities tongue abnormalities	none documented
Pantothenic Acid Helps the body process energy from foods as part of a coenzyme	fatigue insomnia vomiting and other intestinal problems	fluid retention

Nutrient	Function	Deficiency	Toxicity
Biotin	Helps the body process energy and protein from foods as part of a coenzyme; helps to synthesize fat and the storage form of carbohydrate, glycogen	abnormal heartbeat anorexia depression fatigue nausea rash hair loss	none documented
Choline	Helps the body process energy; helps to synthesize other compounds, including neurotransmitters and phospholipids	growth failure kidney failure liver dysfunction, accumulation of fat memory abnormalities	low blood pressure fishy body odor
Vitamin C *Ascorbic Acid*	Formation of collagen needed for scar tissue, bones, and blood vessels; antioxidant; enhances immune function; helps to increase iron absorption from foods; synthesis of thyroid hormone; processing of protein	anemia bleeding gums, loose teeth easily broken bones depression joint pain muscle pain and wasting skin problems susceptibility to infection delayed wound healing	abdominal cramps, diarrhea headache nausea rashes interferes with some medical tests

By attacking the polyunsaturated fats in the cell membrane, the free radical damages the membrane so it can't do its job of protecting the cell. Free radicals also damage other structures inside the cell, including DNA and other molecules such as LDL, cholesterol carriers in the blood. Scientists think that free radicals initiate cancer by causing this damage to the cell and also instigate many of the events leading up to a heart attack.

The production of free radicals occurs during normal metabolism, from exposure to certain dietary components, cigarette smoke, sunlight, smog, or other substances in the environment. Over a lifetime, free radicals may even be responsible for some of the degenerative aspects of aging. Antioxidants grab the free radicals and prevent the damage from spreading to other cells and compounds.

Antioxidants Fight Heart Disease

Exciting research on antioxidants has helped scientists work out theories about how these nutrients protect against heart disease. Most agree that atherosclerosis is most likely the underlying cause of most heart attacks, many strokes, and other diseases of the heart and blood vessels. This process takes place slowly over the years and probably begins in childhood. The linings of the arteries become coated with deposits consisting of cholesterol, fats, and other compounds (called plaques). This used to be called "hardening of the arteries" because it caused the vessels to become rigid and less elastic.

The deposits cause a narrowing and scarring of the arteries, impeding blood flow. Eventually the deposits can grow together, and the artery can close off completely, or a blood clot may form and plug up the narrowed artery. If the blood was on its way to the heart, the result is a heart attack. If the blood was on its way to the brain, a stroke occurs. The blood carries oxygen to these organs, and when the blood can't reach them, this lack of oxygen causes damage and tissue death.

Lipoproteins, which scientists classify by their density, serve as taxicabs in the bloodstream for cholesterol and fats (which aren't soluble in water, and therefore not in blood): VLDL, LDL, and HDL. They're made up of two parts, one which is attracted to water, and another which is attracted to fat. This means that they can pick up fat soluble compounds such as cholesterol with the fat-loving end and travel in a water-based substance such as blood.

Your total blood cholesterol level, which should be 200 or less, is made up of all these lipoproteins. LDL carries cholesterol from the liver where it's made and carries it into the blood, making it more likely that the cholesterol will be deposited in the artery. In contrast, HDL picks up cholesterol in the blood and takes it back to the liver, where it's broken down and disposed of, so HDL is protective. A high level of cholesterol in the blood is considered one of the main risk factors for heart disease because it leads to atherosclerosis. It may be more important, however, to know the ratio of HDL cholesterol to LDL cholesterol rather than just total cholesterol.

This doesn't completely explain a heart attack or stroke. Although high blood cholesterol is a major risk factor, some people with normal levels will have heart attacks and strokes. Some researchers have suggested that the road to a heart attack may be a three-stage process similar to cancer: initiation, progression, and termination. During initiation, the tissue inside the artery suffers an injury. In the progression stage, plaques accumulate in the blood vessel. Finally, in termination, a blood clot forms in the vessel, leading to a heart attack.

Among known risk factors for CVD, some that have been thought to cause injury to the vessels include smoking, hypertension, and the aging process. Studies dating back to the early 1980s indicate that various types of lipid oxidation products, and also LDL cholesterol that has been modified by free radicals, may cause injury. Now researchers believe that these compounds may be involved in all three stages of CVD.

Antioxidants may play a role in CVD prevention by protecting the vulnerable compounds from becoming oxidized. Some of the studies in this area have focused on the essential nutrients with antioxidant functions, such as vitamins C and E and beta-carotene. So far, evidence for vitamin E preventing heart disease is the strongest, mostly because of its function as an antioxidant.

The carotenoids vary as to their antioxidant abilities, and lycopene significantly outpaces both beta-carotene and lutein. Although antioxidant activity seems to be the main reason for their potential role in CVD and cancer prevention, lab studies suggest that, in addition, carotenoids slow down cell proliferation and differentiation, an important step in cancer development. In addition, research results show other biologic activities of the carotenoids including an immunity-boosting effect.

How Cancer Develops

Over the past decades, accumulating environmental problems and more complex lifestyles in concert with an increased life expectancy have forced Americans to focus on cancer as a major health problem. Cancer is now the second leading cause of death in adults and children in the United States, preceded only by CVD in adults and accidents in children. Worldwide, the burden of cancer is equally mind-boggling, with more than 7.6 million new cases every year. Scientists think that up to 80 percent of all cancers are caused by environmental factors and up to 40 percent of those by diet.

The term *cancer* covers a lot of ground and represents a large group of diseases that are highly diverse. But the common thread is the presence of unrestrained growth of cells that began life as normal cells. If you had to name a cause of cancer, it would be the loss of control over normal cell reproduction. Scientists believe that a normal cell transforms into a cancerous cell by going through three stages: initiation, promotion, and progression. In the initiation phase, the genes that control cell reproduction produce a mutation in the cell. Several agents in our environment may trigger the mutation, often by free radical damage: UV light, radiation, chemicals, and viruses. Since the rate of cancer increases with age, researchers also believe that the aging process in cells itself may be involved in cancer cell development.

Even though the tendency for a cell to transform into cancer is initiated, the cell can remain dormant for years. Then, something comes along, a promoter, that activates the dormant cell. This activation by a promoter is called the promotion phase. Promoters change the expression of the genes, or the proteins they make, but scientists haven't figured out the exact nature of this step. The last phase, progression, consists of a sequence of steps. Progression is equally as mysterious, but it probably involves the development of cells into a more malignant state. The final result of the three-stage process are cells that divide in an uncontrolled manner and have the ability to invade nearby structures, eventually traveling far from the original cancer site. This spreading of the cancer from the site of origin is called metastasis.

While the three-stage process seems to put the pieces together, scientists are still uncertain about that very first step, a normal cell developing into cancer. Even that step probably has many complex stages. One thing scientists are fairly clear on is that some aspects of lifestyle are strongly linked to a higher rate of cancer, such as chewing tobacco, smoking, or exposure to chemical toxins. And in a way that is becoming more clear with every genetic study, having certain genes and eating certain foods may provide some protection. This belief is based on the fact that people who are exposed to the same carcinogens don't have the same risk for the disease. One of the most exciting theories involves naturally occurring oxidants and compounds in foods that appear to fight them.

Antioxidants Battle Cancer

Scientists are relatively certain of how free radicals cause cell damage that might lead to cancer, but most of that evidence comes from petri dishes in the lab or in vitro studies. Exactly how this might work in the more complex human animal still needs more study. One of the prominent theories that implicates the oxidation process as the major evildoer is apoptosis, the process of programmed cell death. Scientists now think that free radicals from the environment and our own bodies, and more specifically their subsequent damage, are most likely involved in the first two stages of cancer development, initiation and promotion.

Enough studies over the past several decades have shown that a person's diet can influence the rate of cancer to lead the National Cancer Institute to place a 40 percent figure on that source. But tangled among the weeds of possible carcinogens in food are the latest darlings of the nutrition world, nutritive factors that probably act as anticarcinogens, so that foods serve as both a source of a variety of carcinogens and protective substances. The carcinogens include pesticides, both synthetic and naturally occurring in plants, toxins from microbes, and the result of processing and cooking.

Besides being outright carcinogens, other compounds in food, even some nutrients, may act as promoters in cancer development. A bundle of epidemiologic studies support a strong link between high-fat diets, alcohol, and cancer incidence, with high-fat diets and alcohol use promoting cancer, not actually causing it. In contrast, diets high in fiber, fruits, and vegetables are associated with a lower risk for cancer. As researchers first tried to figure out which nutrients in the protective foods (mostly fruits and vegetables) were the protective compounds, they looked to essential nutrients. The logical choices were vitamins E and C, and vitamin A as beta-carotene. But the more they studied these seemingly simple plant foods, the more complicated it became. An entire world of mysterious pigments and other substances began to emerge, substances previously thought to be merely responsible for putting color on your plate.

As for the vitamins, most studies that consider people's intake have shown that higher intakes of vitamins C and E and carotenoids are linked to lower risk of several types of cancer. For example, a recent review of the studies to date showed that people eating a diet high in fruits and vegetables had a 40 percent lower risk for gastrointestinal and respiratory tract cancer. When scientists pulled out specific vitamins from the diet by computing the amount of each, vitamin C came out on top in cancer protection for those types of cancers. When it came to the types of cancers that are influenced by hormones, such as prostate and breast cancer, carotenoids were most effective, and probably a special one, lycopene, had the edge in prostate cancer.

But to truly prove the connection, intervention studies in which subjects take a supplement of the nutrient would have to turn up positive results. And in this area, the results are mixed at best. So why do the epidemiologic studies show consistent results, but not the intervention studies? Experts have suggested a few possible explanations. It may be that the vitamins and other protective compounds work best together, but, when given without their teammates, they lose their advantage.

Another possibility is that cancer is too complex a disease, developing sometimes over a lifetime, that even the timing of a treatment with vitamins is impossible to hit just right. And maybe it's not just timing the intervention—the studies might not last quite long enough to achieve a protective effect against a disease that takes years to even get going. So for now, the only sure thing is a diet that's high in fruits, vegetables, and other foods linked to lower cancer risk. The American Cancer Society has gone on record with the following advice for different types of cancer.

Breast Cancer

This is a leading cancer site for American women, second only to lung cancer. The studies linking diet to this disease are sometimes hard to interpret because of many influencing factors that are difficult to control, such as circulating hormone levels throughout life, age of menses onset, number of pregnancies and age at first one, duration of breast-feeding, body weight, and exercise. A new area of study involves the phytoestrogen compounds found in soybeans and a few other foods. These compounds are similar to natural estrogen, which studies show is a problem at higher levels. They tend to take its place, but not exert weaker effects, which may protect against breast cancer.

Best Advice

Strictly limit alcohol or avoid it altogether; eat a diet high in fruits and vegetables; eat soy foods; be active; keep weight within a normal range.

Colon and Rectal Cancer

These cancers are the second leading cause of cancer death in both American men and women. They are highly treatable if caught early, but they are easy to miss, often with no symptoms until the cancer has spread.

Best Advice

Eat a diet high in plant foods (fruits, vegetables, whole grains); avoid too much red meat and other animal products; avoid high-fat foods; eat plenty of low-fat dairy products; exercise and stay in a good weight range.

Endometrial Cancer

This cancer of the lining of the uterus is strongly linked to body weight. One factor may be high estrogen levels, so soy foods may be helpful.

Best Advice

Maintain a healthy weight by exercising; eat a healthy diet that includes soybeans.

Lung Cancer

Lung cancer is a major killer of Americans—the leading cause of cancer deaths. Most lung cancers are related to tobacco smoking, probably up to 80 percent, with even passive inhalation recently cited as causing this cancer.

Best Advice

Don't smoke, or if you do, quit; eat a diet high in fruits and vegetables (do the 5-a-Day thing, or more!).

Mouth and Throat Cancer

Smoking is the culprit here, too, but so is chewing and snuffing the stuff. And there is an additive effect when a person uses tobacco and drinks too much alcohol.

Best Advice

Avoid tobacco; go light on alcohol; eat a diet high in fruits and vegetables.

Prostate Cancer

When French president François Mitterand died of this disease, Americans became more aware of its lethal effects. Because it tends to be slow growing, it's another type of cancer that is easy to treat early, but easy to overlook, too. This cancer is influenced by male hormones, much the same as breast cancer and reproductive organ cancers in women. But dietary factors are becoming more important as new studies emerge.

Best Advice

Limit animal foods such as red meats and high-fat dairy products; limit total intake of fat; eat plenty of fruits and vegetables, and especially tomatoes and tomato products (high in lycopene).

Stomach Cancer

Good news on this front—the rate of this cancer is dropping around the world. One causative factor may be a bacteria, *helicobacter pylori*.

Gastritis and ulcers may also be caused by the bacteria, and both diseases increase the risk for stomach cancer. If you have had chronic gastritis or ulcers, you should get checked for the bacteria and, if you come up positive, insist on antibiotic treatment. Diet also shows up as an important factor in most studies.

Best Advice

Do the 5-a-Day!

Do you notice that mantra, 5-a-Day or Better? The fruit and vegetable connection seems to be the strongest for many types of cancer. Figure 4.1 helps you take stock of your intake.

Colorful Characters: Test Your Color and Crunch!

Color and crunch are the keys to those vitamins that fight disease. The best part is that the foods containing these vitamins also contain those mysterious nonnutrients, the phytochemicals that work alongside their more established peers to add punch in clobbering free radicals that cause disease.

The different colors tell you which vitamins and phytochemicals the food contains. Crunch tells you that you're getting plenty of those touchy vitamins destroyed by cooking, such as vitamin C, and crunch usually spells fiber. So pull out your food records again and a palette: Be prepared to be a vitamin artist!

The color groupings in Table 4.3 are mostly fruits and vegetables, with the exception of Dark Brown that covers high-fiber grains. The 5-a-Day recommendation suggests increasing fruit and veggie intake, but five servings is actually a minimum. Figure 4.2 can help you determine your intake of these color groupings. The amount that's right for you depends on how many calories you should be eating, with a range of five to eleven servings that covers a calorie range of 1,200 to 3,000. Go back to Table 2.2 to find your optimal calorie intake.

FIGURE 4.1   An Eye Toward Vitamins: Are You Getting Enough?

Upcoming chapters will describe each vitamin in detail and give you a chance to do a quick checkup on your dietary intake of those vitamins. But for now, let's look at your intake again to try to see if you're covering most of the vitamin bases.

VITAMINS IN YOUR DIET FROM A TO Z

Food Group	*Points*	
Fruits and Vegetables: 5 or more, at least 1 raw daily		
1 dark green/deep orange fruit or vegetable	10	_____
1 citrus fruit or high–vitamin C vegetable (dark, leafy green)	10	_____
other fruits and vegetables, including potatoes for each 2.5		_____
subtotal, possible points of 25		_____
Grains: 4 or more servings of whole grain or enriched		
2 servings of bread, cereal, other grain	10	_____
additional servings, for each	5	_____
subtotal, possible points of 25		_____
Dairy Products: 2 or more servings		
1 serving, for each	12.5	_____
subtotal, possible points of 25		_____
Protein Foods: 2 servings		
2 servings of meat, fish, poultry	12.5	_____
2 servings of legumes	12.5	_____
subtotal, possible points of 25		_____
Grand Total, 100 or more points		_____

SCORE	90–100	Congratulations, it's almost a sure thing that you got all your vitamins!
	89–80	If you are average (height, weight, and so on), you probably got your vitamins.
	79–70	It's still possible you got what you need to prevent deficiencies, but not to fight disease.
	69–60	You probably didn't get even the minimum; try reading this chapter again!

TABLE 4.3   Color Groupings of Fruits and Vegetables

Color Group	*Food Sources*
Dark Green	
These powerhouses contain vitamin A as carotenoids and vitamin C and a special B vitamin, folate, that is new to the heart disease-fighting brigade. The cruciferous vegetables such as broccoli contain many phytochemicals that fight cancer.	broccoli, brussels sprouts, cabbage, collard greens, green peppers, kale, kiwi fruit, mustard greens, romaine lettuce and other dark leaf lettuces, spinach
White and Gentle Yellows	
These foods contain a variety of pigments; some are anthoxanthins, which may act as antioxidants, some are cruciferous, some are excellent sources of vitamin C (generally melons and tropical fruits). Bananas are a good source of B_6; onions and garlic contain allyl sulfides that fight cancer.	bananas, cabbage, cauliflower, corn, garlic, honeydew melon, onions, pineapple
Purple and Deep Red	
These fruits and vegetables are excellent sources of vitamin C, as well as pigments, a group called anthocyanins.	blackberries, blueberries, boysenberries, cherries, cranberries, Flame Tokay grapes, raspberries, red cabbage
Bright Orange/Yellow/Red	
These foods contain a bevy of great nutrients, but they're most notable for containing beta-carotene and other carotenoids. Many of them are excellent sources of vitamin C, especially citrus fruits and those from tropical regions.	apricots, butternut squash, cantaloupe, casaba melon, carrots, mangoes, lemons, oranges, peaches, pumpkin, raspberries, sweet potatoes, yams, strawberries, tangerines, red peppers
Special Pinks and Reds	
These fruits contain lycopene, a phytochemical that scientists have linked to cancer prevention, especially prostate cancer. The list is short so far because scientists still have lots of work to do in analyzing other foods to find this prize-winning pigment.	pink grapefruit, tomatoes, and products made from them (juice, sauce, ketchup), watermelon

TABLE 4.3 (Continued)

Dark Brown

These foods are whole grains that contain their outer covering (bran for fiber) and their inner germ (oil portion). The vitamins they contain include vitamin E and B vitamins linked to heart disease protection.	barley, nuts, oats, wheat germ, whole wheat bread

FIGURE 4.2 **Test Your Color and Crunch**

Points

1) Based on your estimated calorie range as described in Chapter 1, if you met the number of fruit and vegetable servings (range is 5 to 11), give yourself 80 points; if you were one short, give yourself 75 points   _____

2) If you averaged 1 fruit or vegetable from the Dark Green or Bright Orange/Yellow/Red Groups, give yourself 10 points   _____

3) If you averaged 2 servings from the Dark Brown Group, give yourself 10 points, 5 points for 1 serving   _____

4) If you're a man, give yourself 5 points for 1 serving from the Special Pink/Red Group   _____

Grand Total   _____

SCORE	90–100	Fantastic, you should write a book!
	89–80	Great, set your sights on being more choosy with fruits and veggies.
	79–70	You beat out your neighbor (unless he read this book first); go to level 2.
	69–60	Try a bit harder to get in that 5-a-Day or more if you're a big guy!

The Fat Soluble Vitamins: A, E, D, K, and More

A lthough it never quite caught on with some Americans, the extreme low-fat diet craze grabbed a good number of us and still enjoys many faithful adherents. It took nutritionists more time than it should have to point out one of the diet's major flaws: as you cut dietary fat, you reduce the body's ability to absorb fat soluble nutrients.

Of course, the average fat intake could stand to be cut a bit, but some proponents of superlow-fat diets recommend less than 20 percent of calories from fat. Many nutrition researchers believe that below 20 percent there is some reduction in nutrient absorption. And with the excitement surrounding the disease-fighting power of vitamins E and A and vitamin A's cousins, the carotenoids, you want to absorb as much as you can!

Are some Americans cutting back on fat intake so much that it's affecting nutrient absorption? The answer is a resounding yes. A few years back, a young, successful businesswoman came for coun-seling on hypoglycemia, or low blood sugar. She proudly described how she had lost 60 pounds over the past several months by count-ing fat grams. When I asked her about her regimen, she told me she was down to only 15 grams a day. Even on a calorie-restricted diet of about 1,400 calories, that works out to only 10 percent fat—a level that would significantly compromise the body's ability to absorb all fat soluble vitamins. Even leaving aside the exciting research about disease prevention, she probably wasn't getting enough of the fat soluble nutrients to keep up with basic functions.

Although their initial discovery dates back several decades, one or more of the fat soluble vitamins still manages to surprise researchers and jump back into the headlines: "Vitamin A Protects Against Ulcers" or "Vitamin D Fights Colon Cancer." While scien-tists have described these nutrients' basic functions in great detail, much more awaits for creative investigators.

Chapter *Five*

Vitamin A

Although vitamin A, and especially its cousin beta-carotene, is currently a nutrient of popular interest, it's had a long history. Vitamin A was the first of the fat soluble vitamins to be discovered. In 1913, two groups of American researchers unveiled the mystery simultaneously. Both research teams found that animals became sick when fed fat-free diets. The animals failed to grow and suffered a high rate of infection and eye problems, which were relieved by feeding cod liver oil or butterfat.

Ten years later, a Danish researcher reported that a condition in children, xerophthalmia, which can lead to permanent blindness, could be prevented by adding butterfat or oil to their diets. And long before that, history records that the ancient Egyptians were the first to cure night blindness by applying juice squeezed from liver into the eyes of those afflicted. The Greeks subsequently advocated eating liver, in addition to its topical application, for the cure.

The related compound, beta-carotene, arrived on the scene in 1932 when researchers discovered that vegetable foods also possessed vitamin A activity. Closer analysis of vegetables uncovered the class of compounds known as carotenoids, which includes carotene and other yellow pigments. These pigments give the brilliant colors to red and yellow vegetables. Dark green vegetables also contain carotenoids, but the color is masked by the chlorophyl pigment. The same principle keeps leaves from changing color until fall.

Names for vitamin A can be confusing unless you look at the chemical formula. The chemical formula for biologically active vitamin A is an alcohol since it contains a hydroxyl group (oxygen and hydrogen). The name retinol is derived from this alcohol component and vitamin A's function in the retina of the eye. Vitamin A is a generic term for all compounds that have the biological activity of retinol, excluding the carotenoids.

The biological activity of a nutrient tells you about its ability to carry out important functions in the body. Other names and forms include retinyl esters, retinal, retinaldehyde, and retinoic acid. Retinoic acid can carry out some, but not all, of the functions of retinol. The term *retinoid* refers to all forms of retinol both in natural and synthetic forms.

Carotene compounds are called provitamins since they serve as precursors to vitamin A. Humans and animals can't synthesize carotene, but both can convert it to vitamin A in the liver. Of all the carotenoids, beta-carotene gives you the highest amount of active vitamin A, which is why scientists consider it the most important of the carotenoids. In addition, in the average American's diet, beta-carotene supplies almost two-thirds of the vitamin A requirement. More recently, scientists are finding that other carotenoids, like lycopene in tomatoes, offer other health advantages.

Vitamin A in the Body: It's Every Place You Want It to Be

Vitamin A is absorbed into the body in the same way as dietary fat, and, as mentioned, absorption requires some fat. The vitamin enters the bloodstream and goes to the liver for either storage or immediate use. The liver stores 90 percent of the body's vitamin A, and this supply can sustain most people for six months to a year. When cells need vitamin A, the liver makes a carrier called retinol-binding protein (RBP) to transport the vitamin in blood, since vitamin A is fat soluble. And it's a good thing that vitamin A gets around because the jobs it has to do are many and varied: from your toes to your eyes, this nutrient is a must.

One of vitamin A's most important and well-known roles is in maintaining vision. It achieves this through a compound called rhodopsin, also known as visual purple, which enables the eye to adapt to changes in light. When the retina receives light, it splits the rhodopsin molecule into its two constituents, opsin and retinal, or active vitamin A. In the dark, they recombine to form rhodopsin. Every time this reaction occurs, you use up some retinol. This is the reason why one of the first signs of deficiency is night blindness.

Another vital function is in the formation and maintenance of epithelial tissue. These tissues form the body's first line of defense against infections and carcinogens (cancer-causing agents) by serving as barriers to invaders. Epithelial tissues include the skin and membranes lining the eye and mouth cavities, stomach and intestines, lungs, and other organs. Some animal studies show that both retinoids and carotenoids can prevent cancers originating in epithelial tissue.

Vitamin A also plays a critical role in growth and reproduction. Even the earliest studies showed the vitamin's importance by causing growth failure in deficient rats, but scientists have yet to discover how it works. Most think that vitamin A is essential in the growth of soft tissues and bone by affecting protein synthesis, cell division, or cell membrane stability. Female animals who are vitamin A–deficient abort or produce malformed offspring. However it works, normal reproductive function in both sexes depends on adequate vitamin A. Results from human studies show that vitamin A deficiency causes degeneration of the sex glands and eventual sterility—now there's a scary thought!

How Much Is Enough or Too Much?

The amount of vitamin A you need depends on two factors: the foods you eat that contain either active vitamin A, retinol, or its precursors, the carotenoids, and normal functioning of all digestive organs including the liver. For most people, the RDA with its margin of safety, 1,000 RE for men and 800 RE for women, covers these bases. Historically, vitamin A was measured in international units (IU), with one IU being equivalent to the biological activity of 0.6 micrograms of beta-carotene or 0.3 micrograms of retinol.

> ### GREAT DIET IDEAS
>
> 1. Use fresh spinach, romaine lettuce, carrots, and tomatoes in salads.
> 2. Use canned pumpkin in cookies, pies, and desserts.
> 3. Serve baked sweet potatoes in place of baked potatoes for meals.
> 4. Serve fruit salad at breakfast, and include mango, papaya, and cantaloupe.
> 5. Use dried peaches and apricots as a snack.

Retinol Equivalents (RE) were becoming the standard unit for research internationally a few years back. Scientists preferred the RE which is more accurate because it takes into consideration carotenoid conversion. Manufacturers often use IUs, so you still see these units on vitamin labels with one RE the equivalent of 3.33 IUs. But with the increasing awareness of the health importance of various carotenoids independent of their conversion to vitamin A, the use of milligrams (mg) is gaining favor.

Food sources of vitamin A consist of either preformed retinol, which is found only in animal products, or the plant sources of carotene found in dark green, orange, and deep yellow vegetables and some fruits (see Table 5.1 and Fig. 5.1). Food sources offer high concentrations of the vitamin, but some people can still become deficient because the intestinal tract isn't absorbing the nutrient. Poor absorption can be the result of problems in the nutrient-absorbing cells of

TABLE 5.1 Where to Find Vitamin A

Food	Portion Size	Vitamin A (RE)	% of RDI*
Beef liver	3 ounces fried	9,123	1,042
Pumpkin	1 cup canned	5,424	620
Sweet potato	1 whole baked	2,486	284
Carrot	1 whole fresh	2,024	231
Spinach	1 cup cooked	1,474	168
Butternut squash	1 cup baked	1,435	164
Mango	1 medium fresh	806	92
Papaya	1 medium fresh	612	70
Cantaloupe	1 cup fresh	516	59
Turnip greens	½ cup chopped	396	45
Collard greens	1 cup chopped	349	40
Apricot halves	10 halves	253	29
Winter squash	½ cup cubes	235	27
Mustard greens	½ cup chopped	212	24
Broccoli	½ cup frozen	174	20
Parsley	½ cup chopped	156	18
Milk, 2%	8 ounces	140	16
Egg	1 whole fresh	95	11
Cheddar cheese	1 ounce	86	10
Watermelon	1 cup fresh	58	7
Margarine	1 teaspoon, tub type	47	5
Sole/flounder	3 ounces cooked	28	3
Orange	1 medium fresh	26	3
Green beans	½ cup canned	24	3
Corn	½ cup canned	13	2
Apple	1 medium fresh	7	1
Chicken breast	½ roasted skinless	5	0.5
Sirloin steak	3.5 ounces broiled	0	0
Brewer's yeast	1 ounce	0	0
Bread, whole wheat	1 slice	0	0

*Reference Daily Intake

Note: The Food and Drug Administration states that a food providing 10% or more of the recommended amount of a nutrient is a significant source of that nutrient.

FIGURE 5.1   **Check Your Diet for Vitamin A**

Using all of the foods and portion sizes in Table 5.1, "check" your daily diet in the following way:

1. Give yourself 5 (√) for each serving you eat in a day if the food provides more than 100%–80% of the DV.
2. Give yourself 4 (√) for each serving you eat in a day if the food provides 79%–50% of the DV.
3. Give yourself 3 (√) for each serving you eat in a day if the food provides 49%–25% of the DV.
4. Give yourself 2 (√) for each serving you eat in a day if the food provides 24%–10% of the DV.
5. Give yourself 1 (√) for each serving you eat in a day if the food provides 10% of the DV.
6. No (√) for foods providing less than 10% of the DV.

SCORE		
15 or more (√)	Congratulations! Your vitamin A intake is more than adequate. Keep up the good work.
14–10 (√)	You're doing fine. Relax and continue eating a well-balanced diet.
9–5 (√)	You're getting about 50%–100% of the DV for this vitamin.
4–0 (√)	You could use a little help in getting enough of this vitamin. Refer to "great diet ideas" in this section.

the intestines themselves or diseases that affect the intestines. Diseases such as Crohn's and celiac disease cause absorption problems because the absorbing cells become damaged when the disease flares up.

Any disease that affects the digestion or absorption of fat will also reduce the absorption of fat soluble vitamins such as vitamin A. A common example is liver disease, because this organ makes bile, which emulsifies dietary fat so that fat-busting enzymes can digest it. In a similar way, diseases of the pancreas can cause problems with fat and fat soluble nutrients because the pancreas makes the enzymes that digest fats.

Another problem that leads to vitamin A deficiency is when the liver can't convert carotene to active vitamin A, which can occur in liver diseases such as hepatitis. And new research shows that people with diabetes who must use insulin have significantly lower blood levels of both vitamin A and RBP. This might be a concern for those who have low to marginal intakes of vitamin A.

Aside from diseases, researchers know there are some people who just can't absorb beta-carotene because of an unknown genetic defect. These people need to make sure they eat enough foods containing active vitamin A. At the beginning of this section, the problem of very low-fat diets introduced the fat soluble vitamins. The million-dollar question is, "What is too low fat?" Although no one knows the exact answer, and individual variation is important, too, some researchers think that 20 percent fat might be a problem for many people.

Vitamin A deficiency is an international problem, especially in less developed countries. Worldwide, vitamin A deficiency ranks as the second most prevalent nutritional disease behind protein calorie malnutrition. Experts estimate that 1 to 5 million people, mostly infants and children, suffer from the deficiency, and as many as 250,000 become permanently blind as a result. In developing countries, studies have shown that even a marginal vitamin A deficiency leads to higher death rates from respiratory disease and diarrhea, and vitamin A supplementation lowers death and illness rates associated with measles in children.

As you can see from Table 5.1, only foods from animal sources contain active vitamin A. Many people who don't eat dairy products, or take a daily spoonful of cod liver oil, would have a hard time getting enough vitamin A if it weren't for the carotenoids in fruits and vegetables.

FOUR-STAR FOODS

Beef liver
Pumpkin
Sweet potato
Carrot
Spinach
Butternut squash

And remember, too much active vitamin A can be harmful, especially for pregnant women. The arctic explorers who overdosed on polar bear livers died of vitamin A toxicity because of the high content of the vitamin even in chicken livers. You can't get toxic amounts from plant sources because the liver won't convert carotenoids into active vitamin A unless it's needed. Excess amounts of carotenoids will be stored in fat cells accumulating under the skin, and since the compounds are yellow pigments, you might look like you have a serious case of hepatitis!

You can, however, get toxic amounts if dietary intake from animal sources is high. This usually is a result of eating lots of liver, combined with taking vitamin supplements. The toxic level of vitamin A depends on your body size—a 150-pound person would be in trouble if he or she took in about 7,000 RE. Another toxicity concern is for people using a prescription drug, Accutane, for acne. The drug is related to vitamin A, and, like its relative, it is highly toxic.

RESEARCH UPDATE: VITAMIN A AND CANCER

Cervical cancer may be the next frontier in cancer research, based on a recent study. While observing the effects of vitamin A on lab cultures of normal human cells, researchers discovered that the vitamin had surprising effects on cells infected with human papilloma virus (HPV). HPV can convert normal cervical cells into precancerous or malignant ones. However, the presence of large amounts of vitamin A slows, or in some cases stops, cancerous growth in HPV-infected cells.

A recent study from Arizona of 2,297 subjects who had precancerous skin lesions tested whether vitamin A could prevent skin cancer. In this five-year study, researchers assigned subjects to two groups, one receiving a vitamin A supplement and the other a placebo. They found that after almost four years, 526 subjects developed skin cancer, and the vitamin A supplement significantly lowered risk for a specific type of skin cancer, squamous cell cancer.

This is the reason why physicians make sure a person is not pregnant when they prescribe the drug and caution against the patient becoming pregnant while taking it. Another vitamin A relative, Retin-A, also cashes in on the vitamin's role in epithelial tissue by helping to reduce wrinkles.

Interestingly, toxic levels of vitamin A affect the same body areas or functions as does a deficiency. In the digestive tract, deficiency causes diarrhea and so does toxicity, along with other digestive problems. Vitamin A deficiency depresses the immune system, while toxicity stimulates it. And in skin, deficiency plugs up hair follicles with an opaque protein called keratin, and toxicity causes dryness, itching, and the peeling of skin.

Chapter **Six**

Beta-Carotene and the Carotenoids: Vitamin A's First Cousins

W ith all the press this compound continues to receive, it's hard to imagine that beta-carotene didn't arrive on the scene until 1932. That's when researchers figured out that vegetable foods could stand in for animal sources of vitamin A. Initially, beta-carotene was overshadowed by vitamin A because the benefits of this colorful compound were thought to be related to its conversion to vitamin A. While vitamin A may confer a protective effect against epithelial cancers, current research suggests that carotene may protect against other types of cancer and heart disease, as well as boost the immune system.

The Carotenoids

The carotenoids are an eclectic array of compounds, and they seem to be intriguing to everyone. Scientists can't seem to get their research results into print fast enough for a public fascinated by the disease-fighting properties of the carotenoids. Research interest dates back to the first mystery posed by these compounds. Although scientists had been aware that plant foods possessed vitamin A activity, they were stymied by the color of the vegetable tissues when compared to the colorless compound they extracted from liver and animal tissues. Shortly after, they determined that the compound in plant foods was actually a unique substance, quite different from active vitamin A, but one which the body could convert to a colorless form of vitamin A.

Closer analysis of plant tissues uncovered the class of compounds known collectively as carotenoids, a generic term for over 600 compounds (of which the liver can convert about 50 to active vitamin A). Only those carotenoids possessing biologic activity of vitamin A are called provitamin A. They all vary in their ability to convert to active vitamin A, ranging from 20 to 60 percent. Five main carotenoids show up in human blood: alpha-carotene, beta-carotene, lutein, beta-cryptoxanthin, and lycopene. Table 6.1 shows food sources of the various carotenoids with some fruits and vegetables higher in specific carotenoids than others. They exist in two different chemical forms, like mirror images of each other, changing to the other forms when exposed to light, heat, or chemical reaction. One current area of study is whether the two different chemical forms work differently in the body.

The body isn't too efficient in absorbing carotenoids, using only 10 to 30 percent, with most being excreted. As with vitamin A, carotenoids are absorbed along with and the same way as dietary fat. The amount of fat in the diet has a major impact on how much you absorb, as it does for other fat soluble nutrients. One recent study compared carotenoid absorption rate in a diet consisting of 40 percent fat to one with 20 percent fat. The lower-fat diet, a level not uncommon for health-conscious people, showed a significant reduction in absorption. Other factors that can lower carotenoid absorption include fiber intake, smoking, high body weight, and alcohol.

Once inside the intestinal cell, carotenoids can either be converted to vitamin A or be taken up by chylomicrons, the same carriers of the fat you eat, and transported in the bloodstream to the liver. From the liver, carotenoids get back into circulation via other lipoproteins, the same ones that carry cholesterol in the blood.

Lycopene, the main red pigment in some fruits and vegetables, is a form of carotene but, unlike its sister compounds, possesses no vitamin A activity. Scientists are excited, however, about its potential protection against cancer. Tomatoes and tomato products are the best sources of this potent antioxidant, although other fruits and vegetables, such as watermelon and pink grapefruit, can be good sources as well (see Table 6.2).

Ironically, not long after researchers first began studying the compound, they realized that people who frequently eat fast foods get more than their fair share of lycopene. The reason is that when tomatoes are processed for ketchup, tomato paste, pizza sauce, and taco sauce, the compound becomes more concentrated. Interestingly, a recent study suggests that not only does tomato paste contain more lycopene than fresh tomatoes, the compound is more available for human absorption from the paste.

TABLE 6.1   **Food Sources of Selected Carotenoids**

| Food | Carotenoid Content (micrograms) in 3.5-ounce serving | | | |
	Beta-carotene	Alpha-carotene	Lutein	Lycopene
Apricot, canned	1,500	0	2	65
Asparagus, raw	449	0	640	0
Broccoli, cooked	1,300	1	1,800	0
Cantaloupe	3,000	35	0	0
Carrots, raw	7,900	3,600	260	0
Corn, cooked	51	50	780	0
Grapefruit, pink, raw	1,300	0	0	3,362
Green beans, cooked	630	44	740	0
Kiwi fruit, raw	43	0	180	0
Lettuce, iceberg	480	4	1,400	0
Mango	1,300	0	0	0

TABLE 6.2   **Lycopene Content of Various Foods**

Food	Amount in Micrograms
Tomato juice, ½ cup	10,296
Tomato sauce, ½ cup	7,686
Watermelon, 1 cup	6,560
Grapefruit, ½	4,135

But what do these colorful compounds, the cartenoids, do besides subsidize our vitamin A intake that has everyone so excited? Originally known only for serving as vitamin A precursors, current research of carotenoids focuses on other effects in the body. The most important effect is their potent antioxidant activity. Take a few minutes to complete the quiz in Figure 6.1 on cutting your risk for a heart attack. The next sections highlight important new research that may offer clues as to how carotenoids may protect against diseases such as heart disease and cancer.

Beta-Carotene and Immune Function

When most people think about their immune function, they usually think about a body system that protects them against catching the latest flu or cold bug. While this is certainly true, in a similar way the immune system also takes center stage in the body's fight against cancer. This defense plan involves a myriad of antitumor activities, and researchers had theorized that beta-carotene might act as an immunity enhancer by stimulating some of these processes. Immunology experts and nutrition researchers have long known that the body's ability to mount an effective immune response in warding off disease depends on nutritional status and, in some cases, specific nutrients such as zinc. So it wasn't a big leap to consider that individual nutrients might be able to boost immunity.

The immune system is a complex of cells and compounds including lymphocytes, T cells and B cells, specialized liver cells, white blood cells, antibodies, and cells that act like garbage collectors

FIGURE 6.1　Check Out Your Risk for a Heart Attack

This quiz rates your risk for heart disease based on risk factors. If a risk factor applies to you, circle the points associated with that factor. Remember a high score doesn't mean you will have a heart attack; it's simply a red flag that might warrant a checkup with your physician.

Age

if you are age 56 or over	1
if you are age 55 or under	0

Sex

if you are male	1
if you are female	0

Family History

if you have blood relatives who had a heart attack or stroke before age 60	12
if you have blood relatives who have a history of heart disease before age 60	10
if you have blood relatives who had a heart attack or stroke after age 60	6

History

if you have no history of heart disease	0
if you are age 50 or under and had a heart attack, stroke, or heart surgery	20
if you are age 51 or over and have had any of the above	10
if you have none of the above	0
if you have diabetes that was diagnosed before age 40 and you use insulin	10
if you have diabetes that was diagnosed after age 40 and you take insulin or pills	5
if you have diabetes that was diagnosed after age 55 and you control it with diet	3
if you don't have diabetes	0

Smoking

if you smoke 2 packs a day	10
if you smoke 1 to 2 packs a day	6
if you smoke 6 or more cigars or use a pipe every day	6
if you smoke less than 1 pack a day or quit a year or more ago	3
if you never smoked	0

Cholesterol

if your cholesterol is 240 or higher	10
if your cholesterol is 200 to 239	5
if your cholesterol is 199 or lower	0

(Continued)

FIGURE 6.1   (Continued)

Diet—if you consume daily	
red meat; butter; whole milk; cheese; and 7 eggs/week	8
red meat 4 to 6 times per week; margarine; low-fat dairy products, some cheese	4
poultry; fish; little or no red meat; 3 or fewer eggs/week; nonfat dairy	0
Blood Pressure	
if either number is 160 over 100 or higher	10
if either number is 140 over 90, but less than above	5
if both numbers are less than 140 over 90	0
Weight	
if you are 25 pounds overweight (use the formula in Chapter 2)	4
if you are 10 to 24 pounds overweight	2
if you are less than 10 pounds overweight	0
Exercise	
if you do aerobic exercise for more than 20 minutes less than once/week	4
if you do aerobic exercise for more than 20 minutes 1 to 2 times/week	2
if you do aerobic exercise for more than 20 minutes 3 or more times/week	0
Stress	
When waiting, if you are frustrated and easily angered	4
When waiting, if you are impatient and occasionally moody	2
When waiting, if you are comfortable and easygoing	0
Total score	_____

SCORE	36 and above	high risk
	19 to 35	moderate risk
	18 and below	low risk

Source: Adapted from Arizona Heart Institute, Risk Factor Analysis

in the blood, phagocytes. One important type of immune response, cell-mediated immunity (CMI), is involved in resistance to viral and bacterial infections, certain autoimmune diseases, tissue and organ transplant rejection, and some aspects of defense against cancer. The major players of CMI are T cell lymphocytes because they help make antibodies.

The presence of antigens, or foreign particles such as bacteria and viruses, stimulates T cells which initiate CMI. In order for this to occur, a group of compounds called MHC II proteins must be available. The MHC II proteins sit on the surface of some cells and help destroy any type of invader, even cancer cells. We see their importance from studies showing that the degree of immune response is proportional to the level of these MHC II proteins.

Recently, British researchers studied how beta-carotene supplementation affected the immune system. The study included twenty-five men who received either 15 mg of beta-carotene or a placebo for twenty-six days. The researchers measured blood levels of compounds that reflect immune function related to tumor development. Beta-carotene supplements caused increases in blood levels of the MHC II proteins. The beta-carotene supplements also increased the level of tumor necrosis factor, which seeks out cancer cells and helps kill them. And the beneficial effects lasted for several weeks after the subjects stopped taking the beta-carotene.

The researchers suggested that one way beta-carotene boosts immunity is its antioxidant activity, lowering the level of free radicals and protecting lipids in cell membranes from oxidation; they found higher levels of polyunsaturated fatty acids (PUFAs) after beta-carotene supplementation, which supports this theory. And earlier studies showed that free radicals reduce the MHC II protein. Another reason for beta-carotene's immunity-boosting power might be related to its effect on prostaglandins, powerful compounds made by the body that regulate many processes including immune responses. Whichever is correct, it appears that moderate increases in dietary intake of beta-carotene can enhance immune responses.

The only problem with the immune effect is that two studies of beta-carotene in the past few years have linked this carotenoid to an increased risk for lung cancer in smokers. In the first study, from Finland, researchers expected supplements to lower the risk of lung cancer, and their results shocked scientists and consumers alike. The current thinking is that other carotenoids may be responsible for the protective effect, with beta-carotene having the opposite effect in people who smoke. Whatever the reason, the smart consumer will continue eating fruits and vegetables high in all the carotenoids and skip the beta-carotene supplements.

RESEARCH UPDATE: CAROTENOIDS

Cancer: Nearly seventy human studies have documented the association between low intake of beta-carotene and an increased risk of cancer. One study from Johns Hopkins University found that people with low blood levels of beta-carotene had a significantly higher risk of developing lung cancer and melanoma, a deadly form of skin cancer. But remember that not only are smokers the exception, they incur a risk with beta-carotene supplements.

Breast Cancer: Researchers in Boston biopsied breast tissue from women attending a breast clinic between 1989 to 1992 for retinoids, active vitamin A, and carotenoids. They compared the concentrations of retinoids and carotenoids in forty-six cases of breast cancer and sixty-three controls. After adjusting for age, women with higher levels of lutein, lycopene, and beta-carotene had a much lower risk of breast cancer.

Prostate Cancer: Prostate cancer has been on the rise around the globe, and here in the United States, over 370,000 men develop the disease every year. Although treatment options have improved in recent years, the prognosis remains poor, with an annual death toll of 40,000. At the Harvard Medical School, as part of the ongoing Health Professionals Follow-Up Study, researchers interviewed over 51,000 men on their dietary intake of the carotenoids alpha-carotene, lutein, lycopene, and beta-cryptoxanthin. After comparing intakes against cases of prostate cancer, they found that only lycopene intake was associated with lower risk. An analysis of specific food items indicated that of forty-six fruits and vegetables, four were associated with reduced risk: tomato sauce, tomatoes, pizza, and strawberries. Of those foods, only the tomato products contain lycopene. The researchers concluded that their results support current recommendations to increase fruit and vegetable intake to reduce cancer risk. And for prostate cancer prevention, tomato-based foods may confer special protection.

Heart Disease and Stroke: An important study in the early 1990s, EURAMIC, assessed concentrations of carotenoids in subjects from nine European countries to determine if carotenoids lowered risk for heart attacks. Researchers measured carotenoid levels in subjects immediately following a heart attack and performed biopsies within twenty-four hours, which they later compared to healthy controls. People with the highest levels of beta-carotene had the lowest risk.

In the Prospective Basel Study, researchers checked carotene levels in 2,974 subjects. Of the total, 132 died of ischemic heart disease and 31 from stroke. These people had lower plasma carotene concentrations compared to controls, for a 53 percent higher risk for heart disease and stroke.

The Lipid Research Clinics, Coronary Primary Prevention Trial (LRC-CPPT) was a thirteen-year study of 1,899 men with high blood cholesterol, which increased their risk for heart disease. They found that men with higher carotenoid concentrations had significantly lowered risk for heart disease. And risk for death from heart disease was more than double for men in the group with the lowest carotene levels. However, the study did not separate the various carotenoids to determine individual effects.

In addition to heart attacks and strokes, a one-year study demonstrated that people with low blood levels of beta-carotene had more arterial thickening (thickening in a layer of blood vessels which predicts heart disease risk). In 216 of the subjects with high LDL cholesterol, thickening of the arterial wall increased by 0.148 millimeters for each increment lower in blood beta-carotene concentration.

Chapter *Seven*

Vitamin E

W hen scientists discovered vitamin E in 1922, they called it the antisterility vitamin. And since then, vitamin E has been the subject of many studies on a variety of topics. In those early years, much of the research focused on the link between this fat soluble vitamin and reproduction in animals. This led some people to start taking the vitamin in the hopes of increasing sexual potency. As for most vitamins, this kind of thinking didn't pan out. Recently, however, even more exciting connections between vitamin E and a host of diseases are making headlines. Researchers have been studying vitamin E as a key player in the functioning of the immune system, which fights against viruses as well as cancer; protection against heart disease; cataracts and other eye disease; and possible treatment for AIDS, alcoholic liver disease, and Alzheimer's disease.

Vitamin E is actually two distinct groups of compounds comprising at least eight compounds. These include the tocopherols and the tocotrienols (alpha, beta, delta, gamma), and these also exist as mirror images of themselves called isomers, much the same as the carotenoids. The natural form of alpha-tocopherol is known as RRR-alpha-tocopherol (or d-alpha-tocopherol). Adding to the chemical complexity is the fact that synthetic tocopherols, which include some vitamin supplement preparations and foods with added vitamin E, all-rac-alpha-tocopherol (or dl-alpha-tocopherol), give rise to eight more mirror images! And as with the carotenoids, scientists think these isomers may act differently in the body.

Other natural forms include beta-, delta-, and gamma-tocopherols and have small chemical differences compared to their more famous alpha sister. The tocotrienols are similar to the tocopherols, but scientists think that only one of them, only alpha-tocotrienol, appears to have important biologic activity. That important activity is antioxidant ability.

Of all the various forms of vitamin E, alpha-tocopherol is the most powerful antioxidant. And among forms of alpha-tocopherol, the natural vitamin, RRR-alpha-tocopherol, is more potent than the synthetic version, all-rac-alpha-tocopherol. This is one of the few exceptions in which our body can tell the difference between the naturally occurring vitamin and the one made in a lab. But a recent study showed that both were equally effective in preventing oxidation of LDL cholesterol, which scientists think is the reason for vitamin E's protection against heart disease.

The major role of vitamin E is as an antioxidant in body lipids. It's an essential component of all cell membranes where it performs this vital function. Since the lipids in the cell membrane are polyunsaturated and more susceptible to peroxidation, vitamin E sits in the cell membrane and stops oxidation by grabbing the free radicals before they can spread damage. The way antioxidants work is that they become oxidized, sort of sacrificing themselves for the good of the body. And they are rewarded by an ingenious system of teamwork with the other antioxidant nutrients.

Antioxidant nutrients team up to help each other and the cells and compounds they protect in two ways. Fat soluble antioxidants, vitamin E and the carotenoids, protect fat soluble compounds, while the water soluble antioxidant vitamin C provides this service in watery parts of the body, such as blood. Besides covering for each other in different parts of the body, one antioxidant can also revive another after becoming oxidized, which scientists call regeneration. The system reminds you of a baseball game: one antioxidant steps up to the plate after its teammate either strikes out or gets on base. Besides its main function as an antioxidant, vitamin E may be involved in gene expression.

Absorption of vitamin E depends on all the factors involved in dietary fat digestion and is somewhere between 20 and 40 percent. As with all the fat soluble nutrients, vitamin E may be a problem for people who have diseases that cause fat malabsorption. The body absorbs the vitamin less efficiently as you consume higher amounts. After absorption, the liver controls vitamin E's fate and the lipoproteins, LDL and HDL, carry it into the blood. Most of the body's vitamin E is in fat cells.

The RDA for vitamin E is 10 mg and 8 mg for healthy men and women, and the Reference Daily Intake (RDI) on food labels is set at 30 IU for adults. You'll see different units of measure on food products and vitamins, milligrams of alpha-tocopherol equivalents (mg) and also in international units (IU); 1 mg of all-rac-tocophryl acetate is equivalent to 1 IU. Recent dietary intake surveys show that many Americans are not getting enough vitamin E, with intakes well below the RDA. Surveys show that 40 percent of seniors consume significantly less than the RDA for vitamin E. And that's using the RDA as the comparison, which many scientists and nutritionists point out is nowhere near the level used in studies showing protection against diseases.

One problem is that the best sources of vitamin E are plant oils (see Table 7.1). In fact, plants provide the primary source of vitamin E in the diet with soybean, cottonseed, corn, safflower, and wheat germ oil ranking highest on the list. Other food sources include animal products such as eggs and butter, whole vegetables and fruits, and cereals and nuts, which all contain lower amounts of the vitamin in comparison to oils. Our need for vitamin E increases as the amount of polyunsaturated fat in the diet increases. Interestingly, foods that increase the need for vitamin E also provide it. Cutting back on fat makes it difficult to get enough vitamin E.

Do Americans get enough vitamin E (see Fig. 7.1)? Many don't because they don't eat enough of the foods that contain the vitamin, and some may need more of the vitamin than others. A recent study compared vitamin E absorption and transport in young and older people. After giving the subjects a dose of vitamin E and checking blood levels, the results showed that the availability of the vitamin was lower in older people. Another group of people who may need more vitamin E are smokers. Researchers found that smokers had lower levels of essential fatty acids in their red blood cells compared to nonsmokers. When they supplemented the smokers with the vitamin, the level increased to match that of nonsmokers. Researchers believe that red blood cells need a specific ratio of vitamin E to fatty acids to protect the cell membrane against oxidative damage.

> ## GREAT DIET IDEAS
>
> 1. Use wheat germ oil or sunflower oil to make salad dressings or baked goods.
> 2. Serve sweet potato chips instead of potato chips. Slice thin and bake.
> 3. Use peanut butter instead of cream cheese on bagels.
> 4. Put wheat germ on cereal or in yogurt.
> 5. Use sunflower seeds, peanuts, and almonds as a small snack.

So how much vitamin E helps protect against diseases, and are those levels safe? Some studies seem to suggest that it depends on the disease. For heart disease, studies show benefits at 400 IU, and others as low as 200 IU. To boost the immune system, even less will pay off. As for safety, vitamin E appears to be relatively nontoxic, especially compared to other fat soluble vitamins (A and D in particular). Several studies have shown that adults can tolerate up to 800 mg without toxic effect. Most researchers believe that daily supplementation ranging from 100 to 400 mg is safe, and double-blind

TABLE 7.1 **Where to Find Vitamin E**

Food	Portion Size	Vitamin E (mg)	% of DV*
Wheat germ oil	1 tablespoon	20.3	102
Sunflower seeds	1 ounce dry roasted	14.2	71
Mayonnaise	1 tablespoon	11.0	55
Almonds	1 ounce dried	6.7	34
Dried filberts	1 ounce	6.7	34
Sunflower seed oil	1 tablespoon	6.3	32
Sweet potato	1 medium raw	5.9	30
Almond oil	1 tablespoon	5.3	27
Cottonseed oil	1 tablespoon	4.8	24
Safflower oil	1 tablespoon	4.6	23
Wheat germ	¼ cup toasted	4.1	20
Peanut butter	2 tablespoons	3.0	15
Shrimp	3 ounces boiled	3.0	15
Canola oil	1 tablespoon	2.5	13
Asparagus	1 cup cooked	2.4	12
Mango	1 raw medium	2.3	12
Avocado	½ cup	2.3	12
Peanuts	1 ounce dry roasted	2.2	11
Brazil nuts	1 ounce dried	2.1	11
Salmon	3 ounces baked	2.0	10
Corn oil	1 tablespoon	1.9	10
Olive oil	1 tablespoon	1.7	8
Peanut oil	1 tablespoon	1.6	8
Soybean oil	1 tablespoon	1.5	8
Apple	1 fresh medium	1.5	8
Brussels sprouts	1 cup cooked	1.3	7
Spinach	1 cup raw	1.1	5
Macaroni	1 cup cooked	1.0	5
Parsley	1 tablespoon	1.0	5
Pear	1 fresh medium	0.83	4
Cheddar cheese	1 ounce	0.50	3
Broccoli	1 cup raw	0.40	2
Sesame oil	1 tablespoon	0.20	1
Roasted cashews	1 ounce	0.16	<1
Bread, whole wheat	1 slice	0	0

*Daily Values

studies have demonstrated that even larger doses up to 3,200 mg didn't lead to any harmful effects.

A Closer Look at Vitamin E at Work in the Prevention of Heart Disease

Scientists have known for some time that vitamin E is a powerful antioxidant and one of the most effective scavengers of free radicals, not surprising since this appears to be its main job in the cell membrane. And it's this potent antioxidant ability which has riveted attention on fighting disease, especially as researchers add more chronic diseases to the list of those involving free radical

FIGURE 7.1   Check Your Diet for Vitamin E

Using all of the foods and portion sizes in Table 7.1, "check" your diet in the following way:

1. Give yourself 5 (√) for each serving you eat in a day if the food provides less than 100%–80% of the DV.
2. Give yourself 4 (√) for each serving you eat in a day if the food provides 79%–50% of the DV.
3. Give yourself 3 (√) for each serving you eat in a day if the food provides 49%–25% of the DV.
4. Give yourself 2 (√) for each serving you eat in a day if the food provides 24%–10% of the DV.
5. Give yourself 1 (√) for each serving you eat in a day if the food provides 10% of the DV.
6. No (√) for foods providing less than 10% of the DV.

SCORE	15 or more (√)	Congratulations! Your vitamin E intake is more than adequate. Keep up the good work.
	14–10 (√)	You're doing fine. Relax and continue eating a well-balanced diet.
	9–5 (√)	You're getting about 50%–100% of the DV for this vitamin.
	4–0 (√)	You could use a little help in getting enough of this vitamin. Refer to "great diet ideas" in this chapter.

damage. Just this past year, convincing results from a variety of studies led the American Heart Association to name vitamin E as "one of the most noteworthy accomplishments" in the battle against heart disease.

As a major risk factor for heart disease, LDL cholesterol received a lot of attention, but only recently has the antioxidant theory helped to explain why some people with normal LDL still have heart disease. It may well be that when LDL becomes oxidized, it becomes a risk for heart disease. Because of this, researchers have been studying LDL's ability to resist oxidation. In the lab, scientists can make LDL oxidize by adding metal ions, such as iron or copper, much the same as exposure to oxygen in the air oxidizes copper to a green color. Next, they measure levels of key products of oxidation; this tells them how much oxidation is going on. Then, by measuring the time during which no oxidation happens, they know how well LDL is resisting oxidation, a time frame they call the lag phase. From these studies, researchers have learned that each LDL molecule has its own characteristic resistance to oxidation and that antioxidant nutrients can increase LDL's resistance.

Several studies have shown that vitamin E significantly increases LDL oxidation resistance, and this resistance increases as vitamin E content increases. Lag-phase studies are the best evidence so far for the antioxidant teamwork theory. From these, researchers found that vitamin E depends on the involvement of other antioxidants; other fat soluble antioxidants lend a hand within LDL, and water soluble antioxidants help out in the extracellular fluid, which is water based.

Where's the Evidence?

In the early 1990s, an important international study compared blood levels of all the antioxidants in middle-aged men representing sixteen study populations in Europe. The death rate from heart disease among the groups differed by as much as six times. Talk about startling results: in the majority of the groups, two famous risk factors, blood cholesterol and blood pressure, showed no correlation to heart disease death. However, vitamin E levels in the blood showed an important relationship, with higher vitamin E protecting against heart disease death. Comparing all groups, blood pressure and cholesterol were somewhat related to death, but low vitamin E levels proved to be the strongest predictor. In addition, the study also pointed to the teamwork of the antioxidant nutrients, with better antioxidant status associated with a lower heart disease death rate.

A more recent study, the EVA, a population-based study in France, looked at antioxidant status and atherosclerosis among 1,187 men and women aged fifty-nine to seventy-one. The researchers used ultrasound to measure thickening in the major arteries in the neck area and at sites with existing plaques. They also measured blood levels of vitamin E, selenium, carotenoids, and a marker of oxidation called TBARS. The results turned up some interesting gender differences and supported the concept that poor antioxidant status, especially vitamin E, plays a key role in the early stage of atherosclerosis in older people.

FOUR-STAR FOODS

Wheat germ oil
Sunflower seeds
Mayonnaise
Almonds

A similar study by the National Institute of Aging found that seniors who use vitamin E supplements were less likely to die prematurely. The Established Populations for Epidemiologic Studies of the Elderly (EPESE) followed more than 11,000 subjects over the age of sixty-four for nine years to study the effects of vitamins C and E on death rates. People using vitamin E supplements had a 41 percent reduction in risk for heart disease and a 27 percent lower risk for death from any cause.

The Harvard Nurses Health Study followed more than 87,000 women aged thirty-four to fifty-nine for eight years. Those with the highest vitamin E intake, taking a minimum of 100 IU supplement, had a 31 percent lower risk for heart attack. In one of Harvard's earlier studies, the Harvard Health Professionals Study, researchers kept track of over 40,000 men aged forty to seventy-five for four years to see if vitamin E supplements affected the rate of heart disease. Men who took at least 100 IU of vitamin E for two years had a 40 percent reduction in heart disease.

One interesting result of the EVA study was the gender difference: women had higher levels of all antioxidants and TBARS, while men had significantly more artery thickening and more plaques. The scientists believe that women have better antioxidant defenses. As you might expect, the higher the TBARS in men, the greater the number of plaques. In both men and women, those with higher levels of carotenoids had less artery thickening. But after taking into account other CVD risk factors such as body weight and smoking, the relationship was not significant. In contrast, people with higher vitamin E levels had lower artery thickening even after adjusting for other risk factors.

In another recent study, researchers measured TBARS in subjects supplemented with vitamin E. They found that in diabetic patients, who have a higher risk for heart disease, vitamin E supplementation (100 IU per day for three months) significantly lowered TBARS. As an added bonus, vitamin E lowered the blood level of triglyceride, fat in the blood associated with heart disease risk, although it didn't affect cholesterol, HDL, or LDL.

The Iowa Women's Health Study included over 34,000 healthy women to determine the relationship between heart disease mortality and antioxidant intake. After adjusting for age and caloric intake, they reported that women whose vitamin E intake was higher had a lower risk of dying from heart disease. While previous studies found a benefit only from vitamin E supplements, this study showed that even modestly higher dietary intakes lowered risk of heart disease death: 58 percent lower deaths in the highest groups of vitamin E intake of at least 12 IU than in the lowest of less than 5.7 IU per day.

Besides helping to prevent heart disease, vitamin E may help stave off another attack in people who have heart disease. The Cholesterol Lowering Atherosclerosis Study (CLAS) reported that men with a history of bypass surgery who took 100 to 450 IU of vitamin E for two years had less progression, or worsening, of heart lesions compared to a control group.

Another type of surgery to prevent a heart attack is angioplasty, in which surgeons repair a blood vessel that is so clogged up with plaque that blood can't pass through very well, making a heart attack more likely. They insert a needle into the vessel with a tiny balloon attached to the tip. Once the needle is in place, they inflate the balloon, pushing the plaque up against the sides of the vessel, opening it up for blood to pass through smoothly again. One problem with angioplasty is that in many patients the blood vessel clogs up again, a process called restenosis.

A study of 440 angioplasty patients showed that the restenosis rate in patients taking 100 IU of vitamin E per day was 15.8 percent compared to 30 percent for the control group. Interestingly, British scientists reported that angioplasty itself, specifically balloon inflation, causes an "outpouring of free radicals" which increase the likelihood of injury to the vessel and starting the events that lead to restenosis.

Another study of over 2,000 men with heart disease, the Cambridge Heart Antioxidant Trial (CHOAS), reported a 77 percent reduction in heart attacks for men taking 400 or 800 IU of vitamin E for 18 months. CHOAS researchers stated that their findings were "the first from a prospective clinical trial to be consistent with the lipid oxidation theory of human heart disease, and support the use of a high dose of vitamin E to prevent heart attacks in patients with angina and atherosclerosis."

Besides fighting free radicals and protecting LDL, vitamin E may also play a role in another aspect of heart disease, the function of some white blood cells. These white blood cells, monocytes, are key players in the process of atherosclerosis because they stick to the insides of the blood vessel and damage it. In a study at the University of Texas Southwestern Medical Center, researchers gave 1,200 IU of vitamin E to twenty-one healthy subjects for eight weeks to see if the vitamin would affect monocytes. As the amount of vitamin E in the monocytes increased, the release of free radicals dropped and the monocytes were less sticky.

So far, the research is quite convincing: Vitamin E appears to help prevent and possibly treat heart disease in some patients. Of all the claims made for the vitamins these days, the evidence for vitamin E and heart disease is the most compelling. Although a few studies showed a benefit from levels you can get through diet, more of them used higher levels achievable only with a supplement. On the plus side, vitamin E also appears to be one of the safest vitamins.

Vitamin E and Immunity

In addition to destroying free radicals, vitamin E has other antioxidant functions in the body's immune system. The immune system is responsible for warding off foreign invaders entering the body such as infectious bacteria, viruses, and toxins. Oddly enough, one of the ways the immune system fights invaders is by producing free radicals which destroy the invaders. Vitamin E protects the body's cells from any damage the free radicals might cause, even in the line of duty.

In a recent three-year study of 100 healthy men and women, high blood levels of vitamin E were associated with low infection rates. Researchers from Tufts University reported that elderly subjects using varying doses of vitamin E had enhancement immunity. At a dose of 800 IU, elderly subjects had increases in T-cell function. But the researchers also showed stimulation of immune function in subjects using 400 IU over a period of six months.

Another study evaluated the effects of vitamin E supplementation in eighty-eight independent, healthy seniors aged sixty-five and over. After four months, researchers reported that seniors taking 200 mg of vitamin E every day had significant enhancement of several immune function measures compared to the control group: a 65 percent increase in response to skin antigen tests, a sixfold increase in hepatitis B antibodies, and a significant increase in the amount of antibody response to tetanus vaccine. The authors concluded that "our results indicate that a level of vitamin E greater than currently recommended enhances certain clinically relevant indexes of T-cell-mediated function in healthy elderly persons. No adverse effects were observed with vitamin E supplementation."

As for cancer and vitamin E, a recent study from Finland compared women with cancer and healthy controls: Women with the lowest blood levels of vitamin E had a higher risk of cancer than other women. The relationship was strongest for cancers involving epithelial tissue such as the mouth, digestive organs, cervix, and skin. From this study, it appears that low vitamin E intake is a risk factor for cancer in many organs, though not all.

Another recent study from Finland has linked vitamin E with protection against prostate cancer. Researchers were interested in previous epidemiologic studies which suggested that vitamin E and beta-carotene might influence the development of prostate cancer. In a study of over 29,000 male smokers aged fifty to sixty-nine, they gave supplements of both nutrients, separately and together. They randomly assigned subjects to groups of 50 mg of vitamin E, 20 mg of beta-carotene, both agents, or placebo daily for an average of six years. They found 246 new cases and 62 deaths from prostate cancer and a 32 percent reduction in cancer rate among the group taking vitamin E compared to subjects on placebo. In addition, the death rate from prostate cancer was 41 percent lower in the vitamin E group. This study showed a higher risk for prostate cancer among male smokers taking beta-carotene. The authors concluded that long-term vitamin E supplementation significantly reduced both the rate of prostate cancer and death from the disease in male smokers.

Diseases of the Eye

As we age, changes occur in the lens of the eye that may cause several degenerative eye diseases common among the elderly. The first step is a growing cloudiness, or opacity, of the lens, and this leads to the development of cataracts. Researchers believed that oxidative stress was an important cause of the process, and likewise that antioxidant nutrients could help to prevent or at least delay it. A recent study of 410 Finnish men reported that low blood vitamin E levels were significantly associated with increased risk for worsening of lens opacity. When they divided the men into four groups, those in the group with the lowest vitamin E had an almost four times greater risk than men in the group with the highest plasma vitamin E. Cigarette smoking was also an important risk factor for lens opacity.

Although there was strong evidence for a protective role of antioxidant nutrients in the development of cataracts, no one had linked these same nutrients to another eye disease in the elderly that is the leading cause of irreversible blindness, age-related macular degeneration (AMD). In AMD, damage occurs to the small central part of the retina, the macula, and the person loses central vision. The theory behind AMD and the antioxidants suggests that these nutrients prevent the disease by protecting the outer retina, an area containing a high concentration of polyunsaturated fatty acids, which are susceptible to oxidative damage. The antioxidants may also keep the blood vessels that feed the macula healthy.

More proof for antioxidant protection against AMD, this time for carotenoids, comes from the Eye Disease Case-Control Study (EDCCS). Researchers recruited subjects from five major American ophthalmology clinics aged fifty-five to eighty who had a diagnosis of AMD. They found that carotenoid intake reduced AMD risk, and the relationship was linear, meaning that the higher the intake, the lower the risk. People in the group with the highest carotenoid intake had a 43 percent lower risk compared to other subjects.

The study also compared the effects of different carotenoids and found that lutein and zeaxanthin were the most effective in protecting against AMD. The EDCCS authors concluded that "increased intake of foods rich in antioxidants, especially certain carotenoids, may reduce the risk of developing advanced AMD."

Alzheimer's Disease

Not many other words conjure up more dread than Alzheimer's disease (AD). This disease now affects only 5 percent of the U.S. population, but as the number of elderly Americans continues to increase, those affected by Alzheimer's will also increase. New studies are offering hope, however, in the form of antioxidant nutrients. In 1996, an in vitro, or lab, study reported intriguing results which suggested that the degenerative damage associated with AD might be oxidative in nature.

One of the problems in studying AD is that the only way to make a definite diagnosis of AD is by doing an autopsy on a person who has died of the disease. To make the diagnosis, the pathologist looks for a protein, called amyloid, which invades the brain. Besides being a marker for diagnosis, scientists now believe that this protein causes the devastating symptoms of AD.

Based on this theory, researchers of the 1996 in vitro study placed strips of rat blood vessels in solutions containing amyloid. The amyloid interacted with cells in the blood vessels to produce an excess of free radicals, which in turn caused changes in the structure and function of the tissue. The changes included narrowing of the blood vessels, suggesting that this could occur in the brain of AD patients, causing diminished brain function.

Carrying the experiment a step further, they repeated the test but first soaked the blood vessel strips with a powerful antioxidant. When they placed the antioxidant-soaked strips in the amyloid solution, blood vessel strips protected by the antioxidant did not become narrowed. The researchers think that the amyloid in the brains of Alzheimer's patients causes narrowing in the brain's blood vessels by inducing free radical damage. And, more important, antioxidants may prevent the damage that amyloid causes.

The real test for any theory of human disease, however, has to be in humans themselves. A recent study put the antioxidant hypothesis to the test in 341 patients who had moderately severe cases of AD. In this two-year study, researchers used three treatments and a control group who received no treatment: an antioxidant called selegiline (10 mg/day), vitamin E (2,000 IU a day), and both selegiline and vitamin E. They measured the time from the beginning of the study of several outcomes: the occurrence of death, the need for institutionalization, the loss of the ability to perform basic activities of daily living, and the onset of severe dementia. The results were remarkable and supported the antioxidant theory: patients taking selegiline or vitamin E and the combination therapy had major delays in the time to all of the negative outcomes compared with patients in the control group. The authors believe that in patients with moderately severe AD, treatment with selegiline or vitamin E can slow the progression of disease.

Chapter *Eight*

Vitamins D and K

Vitamin D

Vitamin D seems to have been keeping a low profile in the past few years. Recently, however, there has been a resurgence of interest in this fat soluble vitamin related to everything from the obvious, namely osteoporosis, to elusive killers such as high blood pressure, diabetes, and cancer. Along with these exciting possibilities comes new understanding about the exact role of vitamin D in the human body, and a bit of controversy on whether we're getting enough of the vitamin or maybe too much.

The discovery of vitamin D was not the kind that elicited shouts of "Eureka!" from the scientists studying it; it was more of a process, which began in 1919. That year, a researcher named Mellanby showed that cod liver oil and other foods could prevent and even cure rickets, a common disease afflicting many American children. Up to that point, scientists believed that vitamin A, which is also present in the oil, was responsible for this effect. A few years later, McCollum found that if he destroyed the vitamin A in the oil, it could still prevent and cure rickets. And it took twelve more years for scientists to prove that our bodies also produce vitamin D, and that it was chemically different from vitamin D from plant sources.

Some research purists decried the fact that, as they saw it, civilization changed vitamin D from a hormone into a vitamin. But in all fairness to civilization, the chemical compound is a sort of Jekyll and Hyde. If you use the basic definition of a hormone, that being a substance manufactured by one organ of the body affecting another organ or tissue, the vitamin does become a hormone. According to the definition of a vitamin (an essential organic compound required for growth and maintenance of life), vitamin D doesn't quite measure up, since the body can synthesize it. However, most people in the world wouldn't get enough because the body needs adequate exposure to sunlight in order to manufacture it, as illustrated by the American epidemic of rickets seen at the turn of the century before we fortified foods with vitamin D. These considerations generated some debate in scientific circles, but eventually the vitamin camp won out.

Vitamin D: What It Is and What It Does

Of the several forms of vitamin D, almost all begin with a precursor, or provitamin, which needs exposure to ultraviolet radiation (UVR) to eventually become an active form of the vitamin. Plants and bacteria make a precursor, ergosterol, which is converted to ergocalciferol, also called calciferol or D_2. In this form, we can only use a small amount for our vitamin D needs, but food manufacturers start with this source to make an active form of the vitamin and add it to foods to boost vitamin D content of commercial products. How do they do this? The same way other forms become active: exposure to UVR (the manufacturers irradiate ergosterol). After they've irradiated ergosterol and added it to their products, we eat the products and get active vitamin D.

In the human body, the precursor is a sterol compound related to a more infamous sterol, cholesterol. The liver makes the vitamin D precursor, 7-dehydrocholesterol, and releases it into the blood which carries it to the skin. When you're out on a sunny day, the sun's UVR converts the precursor to another form of the vitamin, chole-calciferol or vitamin D_3. But vitamin D_3 still needs a few more finishing touches to become truly active and do the jobs of vitamin D.

The next stop for vitamin D_3 is the liver, where this important organ adds a small chemical group called a hydroxyl. And it takes one more step for the finished product to emerge, a trip to the kidney for the addition of yet another hydroxyl group. Those two hydroxylation reactions are crucial to making active vitamin D, so much so that a person with either liver or kidney disease may easily become deficient. The fancy name for the active vitamin reflects these two steps, with the numbers telling you where on the molecule the hydroxyl groups ended up: 1,25-dihydroxycholecalciferol. If that sounds complicated, it is: The entire process takes up to three days from when the precursor went out to catch some rays. You're not alone if you think it's complex—scientists have found thirty-three more active forms of the vitamin and still don't know what they do!

The main function of vitamin D is in building bone, and more specifically in getting minerals to bone, a process called bone mineralization. Vitamin D has a few tricks to accomplish this, several related to commandeering calcium and phosphorus and boosting their levels in the blood, making them available for bone work. These minerals, and a few others, are important in building bone because they are the key ingredients that make up bone tissue.

One way the vitamin makes more calcium and phosphorus available is by nudging your small intestine to absorb more of these minerals from the foods you eat. And in the best tradition of strategic thinking, vitamin D also attacks the other end: it elbows the kidney to hang on to more minerals instead of dumping them in the urine. So if you absorb more minerals from the foods you eat and you waste less in your urine, blood levels go up and everyone is happy, especially your bones.

But the third of vitamin D's tricks to bump up blood levels seems counterproductive; it increases bone demineralization, or loss of minerals from bone. This paradox becomes clear when you consider how new bone forms. Bones aren't the dead or inflexible structures they appear to be; they are dynamic and constantly changing. In order to make new bone cells, other cells have to be taken apart, a process called bone remodeling (just like the remodeling you might do to your house). So even this seeming loss eventually aids in building bone. And finally, other body parts need calcium, too. This mineral is important in nerve transmission and muscle function; in fact, it's so important that the body can't tolerate even seemingly slight dips in blood levels or these functions are compromised.

Vitamin D Deficiency: What Happens and Who's at Risk?

When you don't have enough vitamin D, the bones lose minerals, a process called demineralization, and become soft and pliable. This softening is called rickets in children, and it causes the legs to bend when carrying the child's weight, leading to permanently bowed legs. In adults, the same condition is called osteomalacia and is most common in women who don't get enough vitamin D or calcium. Osteomalacia can affect bone tissue in the limbs, chest, spine, and pelvis. Other problems, involuntary twitching and muscle spasms, arise as a result of low levels of calcium in the blood and reflect that mineral's role in muscle and nerve function.

The other bone disease is the one that you're probably more familiar with, osteoporosis. In this disease, the person loses bone tissue because of demineralization which makes the bones brittle or porous, leading to fractures. Osteoporosis is responsible for significant disability and chronic pain for millions of Americans: over 28 million Americans either have osteoporosis or are at high risk for its development. The National Osteoporosis Foundation estimates that one in two American women and one in eight men over the age of fifty will suffer an osteoporosis-related fracture in their lifetimes. For reasons yet unclear, 20 percent of the elderly who suffer a hip fracture die within months of the injury. And the monetary cost of osteoporosis is staggering, with estimated costs of nearly $14 billion every year in treatment of osteoporosis-related fractures. With these kinds of statistics, it's not surprising that scientists have turned over every conceivable stone to find the causes of the disease and better treatments.

The questions researchers asked are these: does low vitamin D cause this disease, and can supplements help treat it? Although vitamin D is a key player in bone mineralization by regulating calcium balance, researchers can't agree on the answer to either question. Some studies had shown that osteoporosis patients have lower blood levels of vitamin D compared to healthy people, which suggests a causative association. But other studies have reported no differences in vitamin D blood levels between patients with osteoporosis and controls. On the treatment front, some researchers thought that vitamin D might improve osteoporosis because it increases calcium absorption in the intestine. Again, the studies reported conflicting data, with one study actually demonstrating increased bone loss. Recently there has been some success with combination treatments that include vitamin D and calcium.

If you had asked a nutritionist just a few years ago whether most people get enough vitamin D, he or she probably would have said yes. The nutritionist might have gone on to describe the rickets epidemic at the turn of the century, and how the addition of vitamin D to milk stopped the deficiency in its tracks. He or she might also have pointed to a few groups who continue to be at risk, mostly people living in the northern regions who either don't get enough sunlight or those who have kidney and liver problems. While these risk factors still hold true, a new study suggests that many more Americans may be at risk for vitamin D deficiency.

Several studies within the past decade have shown that elderly people are at risk for several reasons. The most common reason is that the elderly, especially those who are in nursing homes, don't tend to get enough sunlight to convert the precursor in skin to the intermediate compounds needed for active vitamin D. In addition, as we get older, our bodies are less efficient at carrying out the conversion.

Food intake tends to be a problem as well. A person's ability to tolerate the lactose sugar in milk declines with aging, so many elderly people avoid milk, one of the best sources of the vitamin.

Studies have shown that African American children living in urban areas are also at risk for vitamin D deficiency for several reasons. Skin pigmentation affects the conversion reaction in this way: darker skin makes less vitamin D compared to lighter skin given the same exposure to sunlight. Within three hours, the amount of vitamin D available is the same in the darker-skinned person as the lighter-skinned person made in thirty minutes. So it takes more exposure for the darker-skinned person, and in northern regions this may be a problem. The urban setting may mean that parents keep children indoors because of safety concerns. To make matters worse, smog in urban areas filters out the sun's UVR so that less conversion takes place.

> ## GREAT DIET IDEAS
>
> 1. Drink at least two to three 8-ounce glasses of vitamin D–fortified milk each day.
> 2. Receive ten to fifteen minutes of exposure to sunlight three times per week with sunscreen less than 8 SPF (one hour for heavily pigmented skin).
> 3. Use vitamin D–fortified cereals and milk for breakfast.
> 4. As a snack, try pudding made with vitamin D–fortified low-fat milk.
> 5. Use vitamin D–fortified margarine instead of butter.

Nutritionists have known for several years about those high-risk groups, but a 1998 study shows that many Americans may be at risk. Researchers at a Boston hospital reported that among almost 300 hospitalized patients, more than half could be considered vitamin D deficient based on blood tests measuring vitamin D. When they asked patients about their diets, the researchers found that the majority didn't get the recommended amount of the vitamin. Of more concern was the finding that 37 percent of patients who did meet the recommended amount were also deficient. They concluded that not only are most Americans not getting enough vitamin D, the recommendation may not be high enough. Of course, you need to remember that the researchers were studying sick older people, and it's reasonable to assume that illness can affect vitamin D status.

How Much Is Enough and How to Get It

Only animal foods contain active vitamin D, and good sources include liver, butter, fatty fish, and egg yolks (see Table 8.1 and Fig. 8.1). For most Americans, the best sources of vitamin D are foods that are fortified with it. Milk contains 100 IU per cup and constitutes the major source for many segments of the population. Vitamin D was one of the bone health nutrients which received new recommendations last year in Dietary Reference Intakes (DRI). The recommended amount stayed the

FOUR-STAR FOODS
Milk
Fortified cereals
Cod liver oil
Eggs

same for adults, 200 IU, but the committee established new age categories and raised the level for older people (see Table 8.2).

The DRI for vitamin D, like the RDA before it, was difficult to establish because of variability in people's exposure to sunlight. In fact, people in warm, sunny climes regularly exposed to sunlight don't require a dietary source of the vitamin. The use of sunscreens may limit vitamin D conversion from sunlight, but most experts agree that the benefit of preventing skin cancer outweighs this factor. Considering most Americans spend a fair number of hours indoors, especially those who live in northern climates or institutions, a dietary source of vitamin D is essential. If you are seventy-one years old, it might be very difficult to eat enough foods high enough in vitamin D to get 600 IU, which is the equivalent of six cups of milk, or one pound of shrimp, or twenty-one eggs per day! A supplement would seem to be the only way to achieve the recommendation.

TABLE 8.1   **Where to Find Vitamin D**

Food	Portion Size	Vitamin D (mcg)	% of DRI*
Milk, 2%	8 ounces	1.6	33
Corn flakes	1 cup	0.81	16
Cod liver oil	1 tablespoon	0.55	11
Egg	1 whole fresh	0.41	8
Margarine	1 teaspoon, tub type	0.34	7
Frankfurter	1 beef frank	0.18	4
Braunschweiger	1 ounce, tube type	0.15	3
Rice, wild	⅔ cup instant	0.07	1
Rice, white	⅔ cup instant	0.03	<1
Cheddar cheese	1 ounce	0.02	<1

*Dietary Reference Intake

FIGURE 8.1   **Check Your Diet for Vitamin D**

Using all of the foods and portion sizes in Table 8.2, "check" your diet in the following way:

1. Give yourself 5 (√) for each serving you eat in a day if the food provides less than 100%–80% of the DRI.
2. Give yourself 4 (√) for each serving you eat in a day if the food provides 79%–50% of the DRI.
3. Give yourself 3 (√) for each serving you eat in a day if the food provides 49%–25% of the DRI.
4. Give yourself 2 (√) for each serving you eat in a day if the food provides 24%–10% of the DRI.
5. Give yourself 1 (√) for each serving you eat in a day if the food provides 10% of the DRI.
6. No (√) for foods providing less than 10% of the DRI.

FIGURE 8.1   (Continued)

SCORE	15 or more (√)	Congratulations! Your vitamin D intake is more than adequate. Keep up the good work.
	14–10 (√)	You're doing fine. Relax and continue eating a well-balanced diet.
	9–5 (√)	You're getting about 50%–100% of the DRI for this vitamin.
	4–0 (√)	You could use a little help in getting enough of this vitamin. Refer to "great diet ideas" in this chapter.

In an editorial in the *New England Journal of Medicine*, accompanying the Boston hospital study, the author points out the difficulty for elderly people in meeting the DRI through diet alone. He also points out that the study showed 37 percent of patients who did meet the recommended level of intake still had low blood levels of vitamin D, suggesting that the new DRI is too low. Only further studies will confirm if he's right, and there is concern that people might get too much vitamin D.

As with most fat soluble vitamins, vitamin D can be toxic at high levels of intake. The side effects include excess calcium pulled from bone, and high levels of calcium in the blood and urine. The high enough blood level of calcium, hypercalciuria, can cause calcium to be deposited in soft tissue such as the heart and blood vessels. This can result in irreversible damage to the heart and kidneys, leading to death. You don't have to worry about too much sunlight and toxicity because the UVR itself breaks down excess amounts of the vitamin in skin.

The new DRI added a category called tolerable upper intake level (UL) to give consumers an estimate on the highest amount of nutrient intake that would still be safe. For adults of all ages, the UL for vitamin D is 2,000 IU, which is only about three times the DRI for people over age seventy. In a tragic event that demonstrated the vitamin's toxic effects, several people became ill and two died after

TABLE 8.2 **Vitamin D Recommendations**

Age	Recommended IU
19 to 50	200 IU
51 to 70	400 IU
71 and older	600 IU

drinking milk from a dairy that had mistakenly added 500 times the standard amount of vitamin D.

Physicians in Los Angeles recently reported on four patients who were suffering from bone density loss, possibly osteoporosis, and high calcium blood levels. They also had high blood levels of vitamin D, and all four patients had been taking several multivitamin and other dietary supplements, leading the physicians to suspect vitamin D overdose.

RESEARCH UPDATE ON VITAMIN D

Other than the ongoing osteoporosis controversy, the importance of vitamin D to bone health now seems relegated to the vitamin history books. But new studies highlight an impressive array of potential health links for this fat soluble vitamin.

Cardiovascular Disease: New studies suggest that vitamin D may be involved in controlling functions of the heart and blood vessels. Researchers have proposed a role in cardiac muscle contraction and regulation of blood pressure, probably related to vitamin D's role in calcium balance. Calcium has a major role in normal muscle contraction, transmission of nerve impulses, and blood clotting. Several studies have associated problems in calcium metabolism with higher risk for hypertension. One researcher at the University of Alabama recently suggested an association between sunlight exposure and vitamin D conversion to regional differences in rates of high blood pressure, a new hypothesis that awaits testing.

Cancer: Some researchers have suggested that vitamin D may be involved in protection against cancer. This theory is based on the discovery of vitamin D receptor sites in several cancer cells and tumors found in the colon and rectum. Researchers think that the vitamin may inhibit cancer cells' growth and promote their change into nonmalignant cells. Studies of cancer incidence in different regions of the world support the suggestion that vitamin D may be associated with a lower risk for cancer. A recent study from Finland measured blood levels of vitamin D in over 400 men, 146 of whom were later diagnosed with colon or rectal cancer. Finns tend to have low vitamin D status because they live in a cold climate and they don't fortify their food supply with the vitamin. The results showed that many of the men had low vitamin D levels, with 25 percent at or below the cutoff for deficiency. Men with higher levels of vitamin D had lower risk for colon and rectal cancer.

Diabetes: Diabetes is another disease that researchers have been studying with regard to vitamin D. Several studies have reported that the vitamin is important for normal insulin secretion and tolerance to glucose, showing that vitamin D deficiency in animals and humans causes impairment of insulin secretion. Some researchers have suggested that vitamin D's role in diabetes may be related to the presence of receptor sites in the beta cells of the pancreas from which insulin is secreted. Another possible explanation may be related to vitamin D's control of calcium. A study from the Netherlands examined 142 men aged seventy to eighty-eight years to see if blood levels of vitamin D were related to insulin secretion. They used a glucose tolerance test, in which subjects drink a high-glucose solution and their blood and urine are collected for several hours and assessed for how well insulin can deal with the glucose challenge. The researchers found that men with low blood levels of vitamin D tended to have problems tolerating glucose. They suggested that a significant number of cases of Type 2 diabetes, the form that tends to occur in adulthood, might be prevented with adequate vitamin D.

Osteoarthritis: Researchers at Tufts University had hypothesized that low intake and low blood levels of vitamin D might worsen

(Continued)

osteoarthritis and cause the disease to progress. Using data from the large Framingham Heart Study, they examined participants who had knee X rays done between 1983 and 1985, and later between 1992 and 1993, and rated the X rays for the severity of osteoarthritis. The researchers also obtained diet histories to determine the participants' vitamin D intake and blood levels of the vitamin. They considered important variables such as age, gender, body mass index, weight change, injury, physical activity, health status, bone mineral density, and energy intake. The researchers divided the participants into three groups according to both vitamin D intake and blood levels, with a low, middle, and high group for those parameters. The results showed that the risk for osteoarthritis progression increased threefold in participants in the lower and middle groups of vitamin D intake and blood levels of the vitamin. The researchers concluded that low intake and low blood levels of vitamin D increase the risk for progression of osteoarthritis of the knee.

Vitamin K: Wallflower Sister of the Famous Fat Solubles

Vitamin K is the least glamorous of the fat soluble vitamins, waiting in the wings while her sisters take repeated bows on stage for their disease-fighting performances. However, the name gives some indication of its importance; "K" for the Danish word, koagulation, or for Americans, coagulation, its primary function in blood. And if you're unfortunate enough to be bleeding, this is one vitamin you don't want to be missing because it helps your blood to clot to stop the bleeding. So while there doesn't seem to be any intriguing studies linking the vitamin to disease prevention as there are for its fat soluble relatives, our need for it is critical.

Vitamin K was discovered in 1935 by the Danish scientist Dam who recognized it as a compound present in green leaves which prevented hemorrhaging in animals fed a low-fat diet. He later isolated the vitamin from alfalfa in 1939. Vitamin K occurs in nature in two groups of compounds: phylloquinone and menaquinone. A third group is related to the synthetic compound menadione, which is twice as biologically active as the two natural forms. The two natural groups are produced by many bacteria, and fortunately for us humans, the bacteria living in our intestinal tract possess this talent.

Vitamin K's blood-clotting ability is related to its role in the formation of prothrombin and five other proteins that play key roles in the complex process of coagulation. The vitamin is also needed to make proteins present in plasma, bone, and the kidney. Interestingly, when a person becomes deficient in vitamin K, other compounds fill in for these functions. It is the blood-clotting ability that suffers from a deficiency of this vitamin.

The process of blood coagulation involves over forty different substances, some of which promote clotting while others inhibit it. It's the balance of these opposing forces that determines whether blood will clot, and in the normal state, the anticoagulant compounds run the show—a good thing, too, since you'll recall from the discussion on heart attacks, clot formation in the blood is a triggering event. Clotting appears to occur in three stages, which include the formation of prothrombin activator, conversion of prothrombin into thrombin, and conversion of fibrinogen to fibrin threads. Scientists call the process a cascade, much like a large snowball rolling down a hill picking up speed and more snow as it goes along unchecked.

The first step starts with some kind of injury, like the blowout of a blood vessel, which triggers the formation of prothrombin activator. Prothrombin is a protein made by the liver and is normally present in blood. The prothrombin activator, in the presence of calcium, converts prothrombin into thrombin, which acts as an enzyme. The next step involves thrombin acting on another blood protein made by the liver, fibrinogen, to convert it into fibrin. The fibrin compounds form long fibrin threads that form the framework of the clot, like a spider's web, which continues to develop by trapping platelets, blood cells, and plasma.

The threads also stick to the damaged area and the resulting clot prevents blood from flowing past it. Clot formation, or thrombosis, is critical in the case of injury to prevent blood loss. However, this protective mechanism is also responsible for heart attack and stroke when the clot formed after injury to a blood vessel prevents blood from flowing to the heart or brain.

Several compounds, called antagonists, are known to interfere with vitamin K activity because their structure is similar to that of the vitamin. The antagonists compete directly with vitamin K at the site where the vitamin exerts its important effects. Because they don't have the same biological activity, these compounds prevent coagulation, and doctors use several of these for this very purpose, as effective anticoagulants. The first antagonist researchers identified was a substance found in spoiled sweet clover, dicumaral, which is one of many compounds that work against vitamin K. Relatives of dicumaral include warfarin and tromexan, which doctors use to treat blood clots or to thin the blood of people who are at risk for blood clots.

Our Need for Vitamin K

The RDA for vitamin K is 80 and 65 micrograms for adult males and females, respectively. The levels were established based on studies that assessed the amount required to maintain plasma concentrations of prothrombin in the normal range. Food composition tables don't include vitamin K content because scientists haven't yet come up with precise techniques of analyzing foods for the vitamin. The best dietary sources are leafy greens, providing anywhere from 50 to 800 micrograms per 100 grams. Many other foods contain the vitamin, such as dairy products, meats, grains, fruits, and vegetables, but the amount is small at 1 to 50 micrograms for every 100 grams of food (see Table 8.3 and Fig. 8.2).

One of the most important sources of vitamin K comes from our intestinal bacteria, those friendly little organisms that live in the intestine. By itself, this source can't meet the body's total need for the vitamin; experts aren't sure how much is contributed, but some estimate that up to 30 percent of our vitamin K is from this source. Studies which have restricted dietary vitamin K produced alterations in clotting factors. Likewise, people who are on antibiotic therapy for extended periods may become deficient, because in addition to destroying disease-causing bacteria, the drugs also kill the "good" bacteria which produce vitamin K. Studies have shown that even a regimen as brief as five weeks resulted in a significant drop in plasma prothrombin levels, to about 70 percent of normal.

Elderly people in the hospital may be at risk for vitamin K deficiency. Studies have shown that in one such group, 75 percent of patients had low plasma prothrombin levels, which improved after vitamin K treatment. Scientists think that chronic diseases, drug therapy, and poor diet may make the problem worse in people who are ill and weak. In contrast to other vitamins, a recent study proves that the problem isn't related to the effects of aging on vitamin status. In trying to find the best biochemical marker for evaluating vitamin K status, researchers reported that aging didn't much affect it.

FOUR-STAR FOODS

Turnip greens
Beef liver
Spinach
Broccoli

Other high-risk groups include people who have suffered trauma, kidney disease, any disease that causes fat to not be absorbed, and those who are physically debilitated. Other compounds besides antibiotics can interfere with vitamin K. One class of drugs which destroys vitamin K are the sulfas, and chronic use of these drugs is common in people with ulcerative colitis. Even other vitamins can pose problems, with studies dating back to the 1940s showing that megadoses of vitamins A and E could antagonize vitamin K.

Newborn infants get an injection of vitamin K, because they're at risk for vitamin K deficiency for a few interesting reasons. Babies are born with sterile intestinal tracts, free of vitamin K–producing bacteria. It would take up to several weeks for the bacteria to start eking out a living in the intestine. In addition, newborns have low prothrombin levels, which protect them against fatal blood clotting during the stress of birth. But these two facts could conspire against the little tykes in the event of an injury, if they didn't receive that gut-priming dose of the vitamin. There has been some concern that the vitamin K injection newborns receive might be linked to the later development of leukemia. A recent study evaluated hospital records and was unable to clear the vitamin or implicate it, so the jury is still out.

Vitamin K is a fat soluble vitamin, which means that excesses are not excreted too easily, but even large doses given over a long period of time aren't toxic for most people. Two exceptions are infants and pregnant women, who appear to be more sensitive. High doses of the vitamin can cause problems for people who take anticoagulant drugs to prevent clots. In that situation, vitamin K antagonizes the drug and makes it less effective at clot prevention. If you take anticoagulants, you should avoid eating too much of the foods that are high in the vitamin, most notably the nutrient-packed green leafies.

GREAT DIET IDEAS

1. Try turnip greens in soups or as a side dish.
2. Try a main dish stir-fry with broccoli, cauliflower, spinach, carrots, asparagus, and mushrooms.
3. Try spinach, watercress, and tomatoes on sandwiches.
4. Use soybean oil to make salad dressings and serve on a salad of spinach and lettuce with tomatoes and chickpeas.
5. Make coleslaw with low-fat or fat-free dressing and enjoy as an appetizer.

The symptoms of vitamin K overdose include jaundice, or yellowing of the skin and whites of the eyes, destruction of red blood cells, and even brain damage. Some studies have shown that high amounts of the synthetic form, menadione, can destroy red blood cells, causing a disease called hemolytic anemia. However, the form which occurs naturally in foods, phylloquinone, doesn't appear to be toxic.

Compared to what they've done for the reputations of other fat soluble vitamins, researchers haven't uncovered any exciting connections between this humble vitamin and the chronic diseases which plague mankind. But if you "spring a leak," vitamin K will be the most important thing to you aside from a good doctor. As with many of the other vitamins, scientists have yet to figure out every aspect of vitamin K's role in the body, so anything is possible.

TABLE 8.3   Where to Find Vitamin K

Food	Portion Size	Vitamin K (mcg)	% of DV*
Turnip greens	1 cup chopped raw	364	455
Green tea	1 ounce dry	199	249
Spinach	1 cup raw	148	185
Broccoli	1 cup cooked	126	158
Beef liver	3.5 ounces raw	104	104
Cauliflower	1 cup raw	96	120
Soybean oil	1 tablespoon	76	95
Chickpeas	1 ounce dry	74	93
Asparagus	1 cup cooked	69	86
Lentils	1 ounce dry	62	78
Soybeans	1 ounce	53	66
Cabbage	1 cup raw shredded	52	65

(*Continued*)

TABLE 8.3   (Continued)

Food	Portion Size	Vitamin K (mcg)	% of DV*
Mung beans	1 ounce dry	48	60
Green beans	1 cup boiled	44	55
Whole wheat flour	1 cup	36	45
Tomato	1 whole fresh	28	35
Egg	1 whole fresh	25	31
Peas	1 ounce dry	23	29
Wheat bran	1 ounce	23	29
Lettuce, iceberg	1 leaf	22	28
Strawberries	1 cup raw	21	26
Watercress	1 cup chopped	20	25
Oats	1 ounce dry	18	23
Wheat germ	1 ounce	10	13
Carrot	1 medium raw	9	11
Corn oil	1 tablespoon	8	10
Orange	1 fresh medium	7	9
Potato	1 whole baked	6	8
Cucumber	1 cup raw	6	8
Mushrooms	1 cup raw	6	8
Beets	1 cup raw	6	8
Honey	1 tablespoon	5	6
Ground beef	3.5 ounces raw	4	5
Apple	1 fresh medium	4	5
Corn	1 ounce raw	2	3

*Daily Values

FIGURE 8.2   Check Your Diet for Vitamin K

Using all of the foods and portion sizes in Table 8.3, "check" your diet in the ·
following way:

1. Give yourself 5 (√) for each serving you eat in a day if the food provides less
   than 100%–80% of the DV.
2. Give yourself 4 (√) for each serving you eat in a day if the food provides
   79%–50% of the DV.
3. Give yourself 3 (√) for each serving you eat in a day if the food provides
   49%–25% of the DV.
4. Give yourself 2 (√) for each serving you eat in a day if the food provides
   24%–10% of the DV.

FIGURE 8.2   (Continued)

5. Give yourself 1 (√) for each serving you eat in a day if the food provides 10% of the DV.
6. No (√) for foods providing less than 10% of the DV.

SCORE		
	15 or more (√)	Congratulations! Your vitamin K intake is more than adequate. Keep up the good work.
	14–10 (√)	You're doing fine. Relax and continue eating a well-balanced diet.
	9–5 (√)	You're getting about 50%–100% of the DRI for this vitamin.
	4–0 (√)	You could use a little help in getting enough of this vitamin. Refer to "great diet ideas" in this section.

The Water Soluble Vitamins: Not a Lightweight in the Bunch

A fter the heady description of the potent fat soluble vitamins, with important roles such as blood clotting and fighting disease-causing free radicals, you might be tempted to wonder whether the water solubles can measure up. But don't let their team moniker lull you into thinking them lightweights— these vitamins pack a punch! They include vitamin C and the B-complex vitamins, although not all have B-number names.

Vitamin C has been a newsmaker ever since Linus Pauling first proposed it a disease-fighting champ back in the 1970s. Oddly enough, Pauling's early interest in the vitamin's potential for fighting colds has been overshadowed by claims that this humble compound is a powerful warrior stalking free radicals that roam our bloodstreams, wreaking destruction that takes the form of innumerable diseases. As for those busy Bs, some have been grabbing headlines themselves, like the trio B_6, folate, and B_{12}, who have shown their talent for lowering heart attack risk. All of the B vitamins act as part of coenzymes you read about in Section 2, those little helpers that make it possible for us to use food as energy, but each of the B vitamins also has unique functions. Choline, a newcomer to the vitamin list, does not have any known coenzyme functions, but many experts group it with the B vitamins.

In some ways, the B vitamins were the first to be touted as health supplements. Even before vitamin C's notoriety, a stroll down the aisle of any small-town pharmacy would have yielded a bevy of B concoctions with names like "Stress *B* Gone Capsules" or *"B-*Replenisher." A similar stroll today, of course, will be mind-boggling as you try to decipher the claims on literally thousands of health supplements, and the Bs are still there, too. Like most vitamin/health connections, the idea that B vitamins become depleted with a stressful lifestyle is partially based on science; in this case, their coenzyme role. So let's take a stroll ourselves and see what we find down the water soluble aisle.

Chapter *Nine*

Vitamin C

Besides the sniffles, cold and flu season also brings renewed interest in vitamin C, or ascorbic acid as it is also known. Beginning in the 1970s, vitamin C has gained prominence in the research community and among consumers as a nutrient with wide-ranging functions and importance to our health. In 1970, Nobel Prize–winner Linus Pauling spurred public interest in the vitamin with his book, *Vitamin C and the Common Cold*. Up until that time, vitamin C was only notable for its prevention of scurvy, the disease caused by a deficiency of vitamin C, which had been the scourge of sailors over the centuries. Since Pauling's first publication, the controversy has continued and carried into other areas of research about this vitamin. It's not scurvy or the sniffles that has grabbed the national consciousness, but rather the link between vitamin C and diseases involving oxidative damage.

From a historical perspective, man used the vitamin in disease prevention for over 150 years before knowing of its existence. Scientists now think that scurvy accounted for more deaths on long voyages than any other danger sailors faced. In 1753, British physician James Lind seems to have figured it out. He wrote this prescription to prevent scurvy: "Experience indeed sufficiently shows

that as greens or fresh vegetables, with ripe fruits, are the best remedies for it, so they prove the most effectual preservatives against it."
Lind recommended that lemon juice be included in the diet of
sailors, though it wasn't until thirty years later that Captain Cook
followed his advice on a voyage to the Hawaiian Islands and saved
countless lives.

Throughout history, doctors had described the deficiency disease
in ugly detail, but it wasn't until 1928 that the vitamin was isolated
by Szent-Gyorgyi. He named the compound hexuronic acid because
of the six carbon atoms in the molecule. Although vitamin C functions as a vitamin, from a chemical perspective it can be classified
as a carbohydrate because of its structure.

As with many nutrients, our small intestines absorb more vitamin C when we take in less, and less when we take in more, so that
absorption depends mostly on dietary intake. If you are like most
people and your vitamin C intake is anywhere from 30 to 180 mg,
a range which is from half to three times the RDA, you'll absorb 90
percent. If your intake is less than 30 mg, absorption can be as high
as 100 percent, while someone taking vitamin C supplements and
getting more than 1,500 mg will only absorb half. Dividing the total
daily amount of vitamin C into several doses, less than 1 gram each,
increases absorption. Like most vitamins, your body isn't picky
about where you get vitamin C; you'll absorb the same amount
from an orange as you do from a tablet.

Vitamin C Up Close and Personal

Vitamin C has many important roles in the body, most of which
have to do with its antioxidant ability. Since vitamin C is water soluble, it is the most important antioxidant in the watery portions of
the body, while carotenoids and vitamin E work their protection in
the other areas. As an antioxidant, vitamin C acts to become oxidized itself, thereby protecting other compounds inside the water
soluble portion of cells and tissues. In addition, this unique ability

allows the vitamin to be regenerated after oxidation, so it can go on to fight free radicals yet again. As mentioned, vitamins C and E work in concert to protect water and fat soluble areas, with the former sparing vitamin E by reducing the tocopherol radical back to its active form at the cellular membrane separating the water and lipid soluble compartments.

In addition to that role, vitamin C helps the body absorb essential minerals such as iron by donating an electron, also called reducing. Iron in foods is present as the ferric form having two electrons, but it has to pick up an electron and change to the ferrous form for our intestines to absorb it. Vitamin C's donation enhances the absorption of iron, and the increase in absorption is proportional to the amount of vitamin C present in the same meal. Most women of childbearing age and many children have trouble getting enough iron, so vitamin C's help is even more important.

Another crucial function is vitamin C's part in the formation of collagen, a protein which serves as the matrix, a sort of mortar between bricks, on which bone is formed, as well as other types of connective tissue such as tendons and ligaments. Vitamin C teams up with the enzyme that starts the chemical reactions that stabilize the collagen structure. Supporting this role for the vitamin, scientists point to the connective tissue problems which occur when a person develops scurvy.

In a newer role that scientists haven't fully explained, vitamin C appears to be involved in one of the body's critical systems for stopping the action of drugs and toxins, as well as in compounds the body makes, such as hormones. The importance of inactivating toxins is easy to understand, but the same function applied to hormones and prescribed drugs may not be. Hormones exert powerful effects, as do prescription drugs, but if they continue their action unchecked, it could prove harmful or even deadly. Besides fighting free radicals, the vitamin may also work in this way to protect against cancer, by detoxifying carcinogens. Scientists think that vitamin C probably helps out in the chemical reactions that convert various substances to a more water soluble state, making them easy to excrete into the urine. As proof, studies have shown that vitamin C deficiency decreases a person's ability to inactivate and excrete various drugs. And the reverse can occur as well—some drugs, such as oral contraceptives and aspirin, interfere with vitamin C metabolism and lower blood levels of the nutrient. Another interesting interaction relates to heart disease; vitamin C changes the structure of cholesterol in the liver as the first step in excreting it.

Vitamin C is also involved in the synthesis of several key compounds. It speeds up the production of adrenal gland hormones, epinephrine (formerly called adrenalin), and norepinephrine, that act to transmit nerve impulses and are involved in the "fight or flight" response. Vitamin C also helps make the compound carnitine, which helps transport long-chain fatty acids across the cell membrane in order to be oxidized for energy. One more for the list is one of the thyroid hormones which controls metabolic rate. Vitamin C's connection to the thyroid hormone is the reason why physiological stress, such as fever or infection, increases the metabolic rate and hence the need for more vitamin C. It's this relation-

> ## GREAT DIET IDEAS
>
> 1. For snacks, drink fruit and vegetable juices such as orange, tomato, and grapefruit juice.
> 2. Serve stir-fried vegetables as an entrée. Include broccoli, brussels sprouts, green pepper, and cauliflower.
> 3. Regular use of potatoes (mashed, baked, boiled) helps to contribute adequate amounts of vitamin C to the diet.
> 4. Instead of sweets, serve fruit salad as a dessert. Include strawberries, papaya, mango, watermelon, cantaloupe, oranges, and grapefruit.
> 5. For a meatless meal, try fruit and vegetable kabobs. Use green peppers, cherry tomatoes, strawberries, pineapple, broccoli, and papaya.

ship that sparked Dr. Pauling's interest in vitamin C and the common cold.

Pauling recommended taking a dose of vitamin C that exceeds the RDA by 1,600 percent at the first sign of a cold. Studies to prove the connection yielded mixed results, with some showing a modest effect of the vitamin and others showing nothing. The lack of consistent results led most researchers to conclude that Pauling's theories and recommendations were never substantiated. The consensus had been that while vitamin C supplementation doesn't prevent colds, it may lessen the severity and the duration in some people. Recently, researchers did what they call a meta-analysis in which they lump together results from all available studies on the topic and then apply statistics to a cumulative result. The meta-analysis on vitamin C suggests that supplementation reduces the rate of upper respiratory infections by 50 percent in some people, probably those who engage in more strenuous activity.

How Much Do We Need?

You can answer that question by again using that old disclaimer for most nutrients: it depends on who you are. The most recent RDA update increased vitamin C from 45 to 60 mg from the previous level. It also added a new group of people who need to get more vitamin C, people who smoke cigarettes, who should aim for 100 mg every day. The best sources are fruits and vegetables, but not all fruits and veggies are created equal when it comes to this important vitamin (see Table 9.1 and Fig. 9.1). In general, citrus fruits and a few other tropical fruits are the best sources, with one orange and one glass of grapefruit juice surpassing the RDA in one fell swoop. In the vegetable kingdom, your best bets are dark leafy greens and members of the cabbage family, with a mere half cup of broccoli providing more than 90 percent of the vitamin C you need for the entire day.

Even though fruits and vegetables are excellent sources, they also lose significant amounts of vitamin C because of how we tend to store and handle them in food preparation. Because they dissolve in water, most of the water soluble vitamins are touchy, but even within the entire group, some are touchier than others. Vitamin C is sensitive to heat, so cooking vegetables causes a drop in vitamin content, and the longer the food is cooked, the more vitamins you lose. The water soluble nature of vitamin C means that you also lose a significant amount in the water used for preparation and cooking. Try following the tips outlined in Section 2, especially the Southern tradition of recycling the water used to cook green vegetables into soups and stews; this helps reclaim vitamin C lost in the cooking water.

How do Americans stack up against the RDA for vitamin C? Recent dietary intake surveys reported that 20 to 30 percent of American adults consume less than the RDA, and less than 15 percent of children and adults meet the recommended intake. Using certain drugs, many of which people use regularly such as aspirin, can alter the vitamin's metabolism and increase its need. Some scientists are also concerned that, although most people will never develop scurvy, a marginal deficiency of vitamin C may be common. A marginal deficiency of a nutrient won't necessarily cause noticeable symptoms, but it will impair some of the important functions in the body that the nutrient carries out.

> ### FOUR-STAR FOODS
>
> Papaya
> Orange juice
> Brussels sprouts
> Grapefruit juice

A person could develop a marginal deficiency in two ways: not getting enough of the vitamin in the diet, or in situations in which the need for the vitamin is higher. Smoking actually breaks down vitamin C because the smoke contains oxidants, which use up this antioxidant. A variety of conditions that cause stress in the body also increase need: aging, being in a hospital or other institution for prolonged periods, having a chronic disease, alcohol abuse, chronic infections, major operations, extensive burns, exposure to

TABLE 9.1 Where to Find Vitamin C

Food	Portion Size	Vitamin C (mg)	% of DV*
Papaya	1 whole fresh	188	313
Orange juice	1 cup fresh	124	207
Brussels sprouts	1 cup cooked	96	160
Grapefruit juice	1 cup fresh	94	157
Green pepper	1 whole	90	150
Strawberries	1 cup fresh	85	142
Orange	1 fresh medium	80	133
Broccoli	1 cup cooked	74	123
Cauliflower	1 cup cooked	72	120
Cantaloupe	1 cup fresh	68	113
Mango	1 fresh	57	95
Pink grapefruit	½ fresh	47	78
Honeydew melon	1 cup fresh	42	70
Turnip greens	1 cup cooked	40	67
Parsley	½ cup chopped	40	67
Mustard greens	1 cup cooked	36	60
Tomatoes	1 whole canned	36	60
Cabbage	1 cup raw	34	57
Sauerkraut	1 cup canned	34	57
Tomato juice	6 ounces canned	33	55
Raspberries	1 cup fresh	31	52
Butternut squash	1 cup boiled	30	50
Sweet potato	1 baked w/skin	28	47
Baked potato	1 whole	26	43
Pineapple chunks	1 cup fresh	24	40
Asparagus	1 cup cooked	20	33
Watermelon	1 cup fresh	15	25
Apple	1 medium fresh	8	13
Milk, 2%	8 ounces	2	3
Corn	½ cup canned	2	3
Sole/flounder	3 ounces cooked	0	0
Sirloin steak	3.5 ounces broiled	0	0
Bread, whole wheat	1 slice	0	0
Cheddar cheese	1 ounce	0	0
Egg	1 whole fresh	0	0

*Daily Values

FIGURE 9.1   **Check Your Diet for Vitamin C**

Using all of the foods and portion sizes in Table 9.1, "check" your daily diet in the following way:

1. Give yourself 5 (√) for each serving you eat in a day if the food provides less than 100%–80% of the DV.
2. Give yourself 4 (√) for each serving you eat in a day if the food provides 79%–50% of the DV.
3. Give yourself 3 (√) for each serving you eat in a day if the food provides 49%–25% of the DV.
4. Give yourself 2 (√) for each serving you eat in a day if the food provides 24%–10% of the DV.
5. Give yourself 1 (√) for each serving you eat in a day if the food provides 10% of the DV.
6. No (√) for foods providing less than 10% of the DV.

SCORE	15 or more (√)	Congratulations! Your vitamin C intake is more than adequate. Keep up the good work.
	14–10 (√)	You're doing fine. Relax and continue eating a well-balanced diet.
	9–5 (√)	You're getting about 50%–100% of the DV for this vitamin.
	4–0 (√)	You could use a little help in getting enough of this vitamin. Refer to "great diet ideas" in this chapter.

temperature extremes, and intake of toxic heavy metals such as cadmium, lead, and mercury. Of course, pregnant and breast-feeding women have a higher need for vitamin C, with an RDA of 70 and 95, respectively.

It's clear that we fall far short on our intake of this important nutrient, and even those people hitting the RDA may not be on target if some researchers are right about how much we really need. They think that we need more vitamin C than the level the RDA has set. They point to research suggesting a role for the vitamin in fighting diseases such as heart disease and cancer. In a recent and simple study evaluating how the body handles vitamin C, scientists found that a single dose of 200 mg was completely used in human subjects. The authors concluded that based on this and other studies, the RDA for vitamin C should be increased to 200 mg daily.

Supplement Safety

The safety of vitamin C supplementation has been the focus of as much attention as the vitamin C/cold connection. Several studies have attempted to answer the safety question, but, as with other aspects of this vitamin, the verdict is not yet in. One of the potential problems over which the vitamin C naysayers voice concern is that a high intake of vitamin C may cause kidney stones. The theory behind this suggests that vitamin C helps to make a compound, oxalate, that is the main building block of most kidney stones.

More recent and well-controlled studies have concluded that vitamin C does not cause kidney stones. In fact, a recent epidemiologic study showed that vitamin C intake above 1,500 mg was associated with a lower risk for oxalate kidney stones than levels closer to the RDA! The reason for earlier studies showing this connection may have been the result of analytical problems which scientists have since overcome with major advances in technology.

Another purported problem with vitamin C supplements is rebound scurvy. In rebound scurvy, also called conditioned scurvy, high intake of vitamin C might predispose someone to developing the deficiency if they stop taking the supplement. The original theory was based on a case of scurvy in an infant born to a mother who took vitamin C supplements. However, a recent review of the studies appeared in a respected publication, the *American Journal of Clinical Nutrition*, and concluded that the claim for rebound scurvy is "speculative but not substantiated."

So why were people concerned about vitamin C supplement safety to begin with? The answer lies in the numerous studies showing that this nutrient fights heart disease and cancer, but probably at levels well above the RDA. You could achieve high vitamin C levels without supplements, but you'd have to work hard, including hefty portions of citrus fruits and leafy greens on a daily basis.

Although the connection is mostly indirect, based on data from dietary intake studies, the evidence suggests that vitamin C is protective against cancer. Scientists have theorized that vitamin C may work on several fronts to fight cancer. Besides its powerful antioxidant ability, vitamin C may be protective by boosting immune system function including stopping tumor growth and spread through its role in collagen synthesis and by blocking the formation of potent cancer-causing agents called nitrosamines. Fear of these carcinogens caused many Americans to give up hot dogs, which, like other cured meats, contain nitrates and nitrites that convert to nitrosamines in the stomach.

As for heart disease, it's vitamin C's antioxidant punch that is probably responsible for any protective effect, although some studies suggest it may boost HDL levels. But as with cancer, the positive studies to date are mostly population studies and not the more powerful intervention trials. It may well be that vitamin C is only protective against these killers when it works with its teammates. Only more studies will provide the answer, but below are some research highlights.

RESEARCH UPDATE ON VITAMIN C

Heart Disease: A recent study that assessed vitamin C and beta-carotene intake and risk for mortality followed 1,556 middle-aged men during a twenty-four-year period, 522 of whom died during the study. After adjustment for known risk factors, men in the highest group of vitamin C and beta-carotene intake had a 21 percent lower risk for heart disease mortality compared to those with intakes in the lowest intake groups. As for all-cause mortality, the risk was 27 percent lower for men in the group with the highest intake of vitamin C.

A study from Tufts University followed a group of 747 men and women who began the study in 1981 at the age of sixty or older. The group was interesting because of their general good health and knowledge regarding nutrition; as proof, the lowest intake group still had an intake level of 91 mg, well above both the RDA and the typical American intake. Researchers collected three-day food records and blood samples. After twelve years, subjects with plasma vitamin C levels in the middle and highest groups had significantly lower mortality rates, mostly attributable to lower heart disease deaths, than those in the lowest intake group.

In 1995, researchers at the Medical Hospital and Research Center in India studied over 400 patients with suspected heart attacks; half were assigned to a control group and the other half to an intervention group using a special diet. Both groups consumed a low-fat and low-saturated-fat diet, but the intervention group added 400 grams of fruits, vegetables, and legumes to their daily diets. The patients were hospitalized for a minimum of ten days, during which blood plasma levels of antioxidant nutrients (vitamins C and E and beta-carotene), lipid peroxide (a free radical), and enzymes indicative of heart tissue damage were monitored. The results showed that a higher dietary intake of vitamin C increased the amount available in the blood by nearly 80 percent, and the higher intake was associated with a significant reduction in free radicals in the blood. In addition, an enzyme in the blood that indicates the occurrence of a heart attack, lactate dehydrogenase, was significantly lower in the intervention group. The authors concluded that the evidence for an association between plasma vitamin C and acute heart attack is strong.

A small clinical study at the University of Freiburg in Germany reported that vitamin C appears to reverse smoking-induced damage to blood vessels. The connection between smoking and damaging oxidation has been known to researchers for decades; the smoke contains potent oxidants implicated in the development of cancer and heart disease. The researchers injected a compound which causes the artery to dilate into two groups: ten smokers, and ten nonsmokers serving as controls. The compound

(Continued)

was less effective in dilating the smokers' blood vessels than the controls. However, when scientists injected vitamin C before the dilatory compound, the smokers' arteries widened as easily as the nonsmokers' blood vessels, leading the authors to state that the injections "almost completely reverse endothelial dysfunction in chronic smokers."

In addition to its antioxidant ability, vitamin C may exert additional protective effects, one of which earlier research suggested may include raising HDL. The Baltimore Longitudinal Study on Aging reported that older subjects who had higher blood levels of vitamin C also had higher levels of HDL, the cholesterol carrier that takes cholesterol out of circulation and protects against heart attacks and strokes.

Another more recent human study evaluated the relationship between blood levels of vitamin C and lipids, such as cholesterol and trigylceride in 835 men and 1,025 women aged forty-five to seventy-five. They found that higher blood levels of vitamin C were linked to higher levels of HDL and lower vitamin C was linked to higher levels of triglyceride in women, showing a protective role for vitamin C against heart disease risk factors. In men, the connection was weaker and lost statistical significance after adjusting for age and body size. Although the results do not indicate whether the relationship is causal and further studies are needed, they do confirm other evidence that links vitamin C and serum lipids in women.

Cancer: A recent review of vitamin C research showed that for gastrointestinal and respiratory tract cancer, most studies reported at least 40 percent lower risk with diets high in fruits and vegetables. Based on amounts of different nutrients contained in fruits and vegetables, vitamin C was more significantly associated with risk than other nutrients for these cancers.

The Iowa Women's Study assessed antioxidant effectiveness in cancer prevention. After researchers adjusted for age, smoking, and caloric intake, they found that higher intakes of all three antioxidant nutrients, including vitamin C, were linked to lower risk for oral, pharyngeal, esophageal, and stomach cancers.

The study mentioned earlier in Section 2 on multivitamin supplements and colon cancer also showed a positive effect of vitamin C as a single supplement. Researchers at the Fred Hutchinson Cancer Research Center in Seattle reported that vitamin C was associated with an independent risk reduction for colon cancer, although the strongest protection was from vitamin E as a stand-alone supplement.

Immune Function: Vitamin C supplementation improved immune function in a three-year study of patients who had a diagnosis of bronchitis or bronchopneumonia. The randomized, double-blind study assigned fifty-seven subjects to either 200 mg vitamin C or placebo groups. Blood and cell levels of the vitamin were low in the study group before treatment, possibly the result of disease or poor intake. Although patients didn't smoke in the hospital, prior smoking could have caused the reduction in blood vitamin C levels as well. Supplemented patients had better outcomes in terms of clinical progress than the placebo group, which the researchers attributed to vitamin C's role in the immune response to infection. They suggested that vitamin C might neutralize oxidants produced by the patients' own immune systems. And they said that outside the cell, vitamin C may protect against damage that occurs during the inflammatory process by scavenging compounds which may be important in acute respiratory infection.

In another study of vitamin C and immune function, researchers tried to figure out if a critical illness can cause an increase in the generation of free radicals. This British study included sixty-two ICU patients with a range of illnesses and three comparison groups consisting of thirty-four healthy hospital staff members, twenty-one gastritis patients, and twenty-four patients with diabetes. Researchers included these last two groups because free radical production is high in these diseases. They measured blood levels of vitamin C in all four groups and found that plasma vitamin C levels were significantly lower in the ICU patients by an average of 25 percent. Additionally, within the ICU group, the most critically ill patients had the lowest plasma vitamin C levels. Interestingly, of those patients receiving parenteral nutrition (a solution of nutrients infused into the bloodstream), the drop in blood vitamin C was not improved by the solution's standard content of vitamin C, which is 60 mg at the RDA.

(Continued)

Cataracts: A multitude of studies, both experimental and epidemiologic, have shown that vitamin C may protect against cataracts. Studies have shown that the body concentrates vitamin C in the eye lens to a level that is much higher than that of blood. In addition, reports also indicate that the amount of vitamin C in the lens changes as dietary intake of the vitamin changes. In a recent study, 247 women aged fifty-six to seventy-one had eye exams to find the beginnings of cataracts, early lens opacities. Women who used vitamin C supplements for ten years or more had a 77 percent lower risk for early lens opacities and an 83 percent lower risk for more advanced opacities. The authors concluded that the results of their study support other evidence that links vitamin C supplements to lower risk for cataracts.

Chapter **Ten**

Vitamins B₁ (Thiamin), B₂ (Riboflavin), and B₃ (Niacin)

Vitamin B₁ (Thiamin)

While Americans are continuing their love affair with vitamins, most people don't think much about thiamin. For many years, the biggest controversy about this vitamin had been how to spell it— with an "e" on the end or without. But some of our ancestors weren't so fortunate and succumbed in large numbers to the ravages of beriberi, the traditional name for thiamin deficiency.

Scientists first isolated thiamin in 1926, but centuries before this, the deficiency disease ran rampant throughout the Far East. The earliest mention of what was most certainly thiamin deficiency was in *Neiching*, a Chinese medical book, dating back to 2697 B.C.E. Beriberi means "I can't, I can't" in Sinhalese and earned its name because of a peculiar head movement associated with the nerve damage accompanying the disease. In a nutrition coup similar to that for vitamin C, a nineteenth-century surgeon in the Japanese navy found that adding meat and whole grains to the usual navy rations dramatically reduced the incidence of beriberi among sailors. Although it's tragic that thousands of sailors died, those long sea voyages were the perfect vehicle for helping scientists to learn about vitamins.

Fifteen years later, a Dutch prison physician discovered a similar connection. Prisoners who were fed polished rice, that had lost most of its thiamin along with the rice bran, developed beriberi. The "scraps" of rice bran, in turn, were used as chicken feed. He noticed that when the chickens ate the same rice as the prisoners, they also developed the disease. More important, he discovered that by feeding the chickens rice bran, the disease was cured.

When it was isolated in the early 1920s, it was named "the B vitamin." Later, nutrition researchers had to assign numbers to the other B vitamins, which they discovered shortly thereafter, and figured out that what was thought to be one nutrient were actually several. Once they named it, it was easy to learn what the vitamin does in the body. The major role of thiamin is as a coenzyme, as are the other B vitamins, that helps release energy from carbohydrate in the foods you eat. Thiamin is also involved in nerve transmission, sitting on the nerve cell membrane, and helps orchestrate nerve impulses and movement in muscles as a result.

The symptoms of thiamin deficiency dramatically show its importance in nerve function, although the specific clinical picture depends on the person's age. Beriberi can either be wet, referring to water retention, or dry, characterized by muscle wasting. Dry

GREAT DIET IDEAS

1. Include lean pork (tenderloin, loin chops, lean ham, Canadian bacon, and loin roast) in your weekly menus.
2. Make economical soups and salads that contain green peas, black beans, split peas, black-eyed peas, and kidney beans.
3. Use enriched macaroni, pasta, and bread products.
4. Serve oatmeal or fortified cereals for breakfast (they contain approximately 25 percent of the DRI for thiamin).
5. Use boiled or baked squash as a side dish.

beriberi strikes the nervous system and induces spasms and uncontrolled movement, and wet beriberi mostly affects the heart. The deficiency is most common in infants between the ages of two and three months. Thiamin-deficient babies with wet beriberi cry in loud piercing tones, turn blue, vomit, and have trouble breathing. The heart becomes enlarged, and death can follow within hours unless they receive a dose of thiamin. In infants with dry beriberi, crying ranges from hoarseness to no sound at all, and nerve damage shows up as purposeless movement of the hands and arms.

Wet beriberi in adults causes fluid retention, rapid heartbeat, heart enlargement, and eventual congestive heart failure. Adults can also develop a type of beriberi that affects the brain and nervous system, Wernicke-Korsakoff syndrome. Although each of those two words can be two separate disorders, they often appear together, especially in cases of alcohol abuse. The symptoms include mental confusion, unsteady gait, and significant memory dysfunction. Scientists now believe that some people may have a subclinical deficiency, showing no overt signs, only general symptoms such as irritability, headaches, and fatigue.

> ### FOUR-STAR FOODS
> ---
> Brewer's yeast
> Pork chops
> Ham
> Green peas

How Much Do We Need?

The new DRI for thiamin is lower than the 1989 RDA at 1.2 mg for men and 1.1 mg for women. Because of its role in energy metabolism, the requirement is based on caloric intake. So the more calories you take in, the more thiamin you need as well, and this is true for all B vitamins that help process energy. Although it's widely distributed in the food supply through grain products, excellent sources include organ meats, pork, brewer's yeast, and whole grains (see Table 10.1 and Fig. 9.1). Thiamin is one of the safest vitamins, with no reports of side effects even at high doses of 500 mg daily over a month-long period.

Like other B vitamins, thiamin is lost in the flour milling process as the outer covering and bran are removed. To combat nutrient deficiencies, several decades ago the government passed legislation, the Flour Enrichment Act, mandating the addition of thiamin, riboflavin, niacin, and iron to flour. So the term *enriched grain products* refers to cereals and baked goods made from flour that has this added quartet of nutrients. Of course, if you eat the whole grain product, you get the added bonus of bran and the germ inside the grain head. The germ contains even more vitamins and minerals and, of special interest, fat soluble nutrients such as vitamin E.

Some other ways of losing thiamin include the practice of adding sodium bicarbonate, baking soda, to green beans and peas to keep the pretty green color during cooking, and to dried beans and peas to soften their skins. The baking soda inactivates the thiamin, so it no longer can carry out its functions in the body. High cooking temperatures also destroy the vitamin, with temperatures used to cook meats, vegetables, and grain products causing losses of up to 50 percent. Just like its other water soluble relatives, thiamin will be lost in cooking water that you pour down the drain. One storage technique that doesn't affect this sensitive vitamin is freezing.

Several compounds that occur naturally in foods can interfere with thiamin, and they're important enough to have earned a name for this action: antithiamin factors (ATF). Some of the foods that contain ATF include freshwater fish guts, shellfish, ferns, tea, and some vegetables. Scientists have reported cases of thiamin deficiency caused by excessive intake of tea and coffee in combination with a diet that's not high in thiamin to start with. The minerals calcium and magnesium interact with tannin compounds in tea, coffee, nuts, and wine to compound the thiamin interference. But there are some helpers as well, with vitamin C boosting thiamin status and the acid in fruits and vegetables protecting against the action of the minerals.

Chronic alcoholics are likely to become deficient for several reasons. One obvious reason relates to the poor diet that is typical in chronic alcoholism. Other factors are more complex and involve

TABLE 10.1 Where to Find Vitamin B₁ (Thiamin)

Food	Portion Size	Thiamin (mg)	% of DRI* Women	% of DRI* Men
Brewer's yeast	1 ounce	4.43	403	369
Pork chop	3.5 ounces roasted	0.91	83	76
Ham	3.5 ounces cooked	0.78	71	65
Green peas	1 cup cooked	0.42	38	35
Canadian bacon	2 pieces cooked	0.38	35	32
Corn flakes	1 cup	0.38	35	32
Split peas	1 cup cooked	0.37	34	31
Macaroni, enriched	1 cup cooked	0.29	26	24
Kidney beans	1 cup canned	0.27	25	23
Oatmeal	1 cup cooked	0.26	24	22
Millet	1 cup cooked	0.25	23	21
Acorn squash	1 cup boiled	0.24	22	20
Baked potato	1 whole	0.22	20	18
Asparagus	1 cup cooked	0.22	20	18
Peanuts	1 ounce dry, unsalted	0.19	17	16
Black-eyed peas	1 cup cooked	0.17	15	14
Watermelon	1 cup fresh	0.13	12	11
Sirloin steak	3.5 ounces broiled	0.13	12	11
Honeydew melon	1 cup fresh	0.13	12	11
Orange	1 fresh medium	0.12	11	10
Winter squash	1 cup baked	0.12	11	10
Tofu	½ cup	0.10	9	8
Milk, 2%	8 ounces	0.10	9	8
Green beans	1 cup cooked	0.10	9	8
Broccoli	1 cup cooked	0.10	9	8
Bread, whole wheat	1 slice	0.09	8	8
Sole/flounder	3 ounces cooked	0.08	7	7

(Continued)

TABLE 10.1   (Continued)

Food	Portion Size	Thiamin (mg)	% of DRI* Women	% of DRI* Men
Cauliflower	1 cup cooked	0.08	7	7
Tomato	1 whole raw	0.07	6	6
Cantaloupe	1 cup fresh	0.06	5	5
Oysters	1 cup raw	0.06	5	5
Sunflower seeds	¼ cup, dry roasted	0.03	3	2.5
Bean sprouts	1 cup fresh	0.03	3	2.5
Apple	1 fresh medium	0.02	2	2

*Dietary Reference Intake

FIGURE 10.1   Check Your Diet for Vitamin B₁ (Thiamin)

Using all of the foods and portion sizes in Table 10.1, "check" your daily diet in the following way:

1. Give yourself 5 (√) for each serving you eat in a day if the food provides less than 100%–80% of the DRI.
2. Give yourself 4 (√) for each serving you eat in a day if the food provides 79%–50% of the DRI.
3. Give yourself 3 (√) for each serving you eat in a day if the food provides 49%–25% of the DRI.
4. Give yourself 2 (√) for each serving you eat in a day if the food provides 24%–10% of the DRI.
5. Give yourself 1 (√) for each serving you eat in a day if the food provides 10% of the DRI.
6. No (√) for foods providing less than 10% of the DRI.

SCORE	15 or more (√)	Congratulations! Your thiamin intake is more than adequate. Keep up the good work.
	14–10 (√)	You're doing fine. Relax and continue eating a well-balanced diet.
	9–5 (√)	You're getting about 50%–100% of the DRI for this vitamin.
	4–0 (√)	You could use a little help in getting enough of this vitamin. Refer to "great diet ideas" in this section.

various aspects of thiamin absorption, which is decreased in alcoholism, and thiamin metabolism. The vitamin is necessary for alcohol metabolism, and with excessive alcohol ingestion, this takes precedence over other metabolic functions in which thiamin is involved.

Some other groups may also be at risk for thiamin deficiency. Surveys of vitamin intake in the United States show that the average woman's intake barely met the previous RDA. And breast-fed babies whose mothers are thiamin deficient are also at risk for beriberi. At the other end of the age spectrum, the elderly may be vulnerable as well. They often rely on highly processed foods which are easy to prepare, but because thiamin is easily destroyed by processing heat, their intake of the vitamin may be lower than they need. Any condition that increases the need for thiamin can cause a deficiency, especially if intake is less than ideal. Some of these include strenuous physical activity, pregnancy and lactation, fever, and even adolescence.

One special situation is people who may have a moderate deficiency (not enough for dramatic symptoms) and eat a high-carbohydrate diet. Human studies from the 1940s showed that when moderately deficient subjects were given a dose of glucose, blood levels of lactic and pyruvic acids went up. High levels of these compounds mean that the body is not converting carbohydrate to energy as efficiently as it should.

In a similar vein, other studies reported that glucose loading increased liver and heart glycogen levels, the storage form of carbohydrate. Research has shown that carbohydrate loading can precipitate thiamin-induced nerve damage, and physical activity of as little as one minute of exercise after glucose loading increases pyruvic and lactic acids in thiamin-depleted subjects. This may be of practical concern to athletes who do the popular carbohydrate loading before an event and may not be getting quite enough thiamin in their diets.

Most Americans get enough thiamin, thanks mostly to the Flour Enrichment Act, but both intake surveys and clinical trials have shown that some people are vulnerable to a deficiency of this important nutrient. Thiamin may have been the first B vitamin discovered, but this vitamin's story is continuing. And for the spelling enthusiasts, the accepted American spelling is without an "e" on the end. Following are a few highlights of recent thiamin research.

RESEARCH UPDATE ON THIAMIN

Thiamin Functions: Scientists have discovered special compounds, tissue factors, that limit how much thiamin can become active in the body—sort of like how your computer printer has a buffer that holds the text you want until it's ready to print. They also believe that thiamin may be involved in the pancreas's role in making insulin.

Dialysis Patients: People with kidney disease who need dialysis, blood filtering done by machine, often have several nutrient deficiencies. A recent study reviewed thiamin and other B vitamins in twenty-one dialysis patients. The patients were low in these nutrients, and in an effort to improve their status, researchers provided diet counseling for eight weeks. As a result, some nutrition parameters improved, but others couldn't be improved because the dialysis requires a special and limited diet. The authors concluded that dialysis patients need regular supplementation of B vitamins.

Colon Cancer: Epidemiologic studies have shown that plant foods are linked to lower risk for colon cancer. A recent study tried to figure out which nutrients in the plant foods were responsible for the protective effect. They compared over 4,000 people from northern California, Utah, and the "Twin Cities" area of Minnesota; roughly half developed colon cancer and half didn't. Plant foods are good sources of thiamin, vitamin B_6, and niacin. In women only, these nutrients seemed to be protective against colon cancer.

Head Injuries: Doctors give alcoholic patients a dose of thiamin to prevent Wernicke-Korsakoff syndrome, which can result in coma. To determine how these people, and others with head injuries, are treated and the results, a Scottish study looked at these patients. They found that only 20.6 percent of patients with head injuries received thiamin, with just over half, 56.1 percent, of those categorized as alcoholic receiving this treatment. In the patients who did receive thiamin, the dose and duration were inadequate in most cases. The authors suggest that doctors should give thiamin to head injury patients at risk of Wernicke-Korsakoff syndrome to prevent additional damage to the injured brain.

Thiamin Status in Breast-feeding Women: A recent Canadian study evaluated the nutrient intakes of women who are breast-feeding, an important consideration since nutrients pass into the breast milk to the infant. Researchers interviewed 183 women breast-feeding at three months postpartum; the women lived in low-income communities. The results showed that most women didn't get the calories they needed to breast-feed, and they didn't meet the 1989 RDA for thiamin and several other nutrients. The authors concluded that low-income women who are breast-feeding are at high risk of energy and nutrient inadequacies, including thiamin.

Thiamin Status in the Elderly: This study examined subclinical thiamin deficiency in the elderly to learn if treating the patients with thiamin had any significant impact on health. About 18 percent of the patients had a low level of thiamin on one occasion when tested, and another 16 percent had low levels on more than one test. All the patients received a thiamin supplement, but only those with low levels on two occasions had measurable improvements in health. In those patients, both blood pressure and weight were lower after treatment with the vitamin.

Vitamin B$_2$ (Riboflavin)

As with several of the B vitamins, riboflavin caused quite a stir when scientists first discovered it, but this essential nutrient was soon relegated to the back of the closet as more famous relatives arrived on the scene. Riboflavin makes its presence felt from time to time or, more accurately, its absence, when manufacturers and consumers fail to handle it with care.

The alias for this nutrient, B_2, helps to explain its second-rate status. As mentioned in the thiamin section, the disease beriberi was a scourge around the world for centuries, causing damage to the nervous and cardiovascular systems and many deaths. The discovery by a Japanese navy surgeon and the Dutch scientist Eijkmann that certain foods could prevent and cure beriberi seemed to solve the mystery of the disease, and when scientists isolated the nutrient in the late 1920s, they thought they'd discovered the antiberiberi factor.

It didn't take long before they realized their error—the antiberiberi factor was actually two different compounds. This finally led to the discovery of riboflavin, which was labeled B_2 in England and vitamin G in the United States. Later, more B vitamins joined the list, some with ascending numbers. Riboflavin's fluorescent orange-yellow color helped the researchers make their discovery, because it was readily detectable in food extracts. The bright color also gave scientists some help with the vitamin's other name: *flavus* is yellow in Latin. The other part of its name comes from a sugar the vitamin contains, ribitol.

The vitamin is a part of two different coenzymes in the body which, in turn, function in many enzyme systems. Some of the enzyme systems include those involved in energy production and the

GREAT DIET IDEAS

1. A bowl of corn flakes with 8 ounces of milk provides 75 percent of the DRI of riboflavin for women.
2. Use yogurt as a snack and as a dip for fruits and vegetables.
3. Mushrooms are a very low-calorie source of riboflavin. Use them in pizza, salads, or stir-frys.
4. Use low-fat cottage or ricotta cheeses in lasagna, ravioli, or other main-dish meals.
5. Include four glasses of low-fat milk daily to achieve approximately 100 percent of the DRI for riboflavin.

conversion of the amino acid tryptophan to the B vitamin niacin, a handy reaction if you're short of niacin. Dietary sources of riboflavin include meats, poultry, fish, and particularly dairy products (see Table 10.2 and Fig. 10.2). Whole grain and enriched products supply a large amount of riboflavin to most Americans. Other good sources of riboflavin are leafy green vegetables, although because of its solubility in water, significant amounts are lost in the water used to cook these vegetables. By the same principle, excess amounts are readily excreted in the urine, making it a relatively safe vitamin. Unlike others of its ilk, the vitamin is stable to heat, but it is sensitive to light.

The new DRI for riboflavin is 1.3 mg and 1.1 mg for women and men, respectively. Dietary intake surveys show that most Americans are meeting the recommended levels. Around the world, riboflavin deficiency is common, although it usually occurs in combination with deficiencies of other B vitamins. Signs of the deficiency include fluid retention, sore throat, and inflammation of the tongue and mouth. People who have abnormal hormone levels, especially thyroid hormone, may not metabolize the vitamin properly, and some drugs, including oral contraceptives and barbiturates, can cause problems.

Some groups of Americans may also be at risk for riboflavin deficiency, including athletes, women, alcoholics, and people who don't eat dairy products. Athletes have a greater energy demand and this uses up riboflavin. Women and alcoholics tend to have a less nutrient-dense diet and are more likely to avoid milk. Since milk and dairy products are the best source, eliminating them may lead to a riboflavin deficiency.

Public attention began less than ten years ago, when studies reported major losses of riboflavin from milk in opaque plastic containers. Although scientists had known for decades that riboflavin is sensitive to light, no one gave the new milk cartons much thought when they replaced the old-fashioned paper cartons. Because dairy products are the most concentrated source of the vitamin in the U.S. food supply, however, when the concern surfaced, it seemed

TABLE 10.2 Where to Find Vitamin B₂ (Riboflavin)

Food	Portion Size	Riboflavin	% of DRI* Women	% of DRI* Men
Brewer's yeast	1 tablespoon	1.21	110	93
Yogurt, low fat	1 cup	0.51	46	39
Mushrooms	1 cup cooked	0.46	42	35
Ricotta cheese, part skim	1 cup	0.46	42	35
Braunschweiger	1 ounce, tube type	0.43	39	33
Corn flakes	1 cup	0.43	39	33
Cottage cheese, low fat	1 cup	0.42	38	32
Beet greens	1 cup cooked	0.42	38	32
Milk, 2%	8 ounces	0.40	36	31
Buttermilk	1 cup	0.38	35	29
Goat's milk	1 cup	0.34	31	26
Sirloin steak	3.5 ounces, broiled	0.29	26	22
Peach halves	10 dried	0.28	25	22
Pork chop	3.5 ounces roasted	0.26	24	20
Ground beef	3.5 ounces lean baked	0.24	22	18
Black-eyed peas	1 cup cooked	0.24	22	18
Kidney beans	1 cup canned	0.23	21	18
Asparagus	1 cup cooked	0.22	20	17
Almonds	1 ounce whole dried	0.22	20	17
Oysters	3 ounces raw	0.20	18	15
Ham	3.5 ounces cooked	0.19	17	15
Turkey	3.5 ounces skinless	0.18	16	14
Soy milk	1 cup	0.17	15	13
Broccoli	1 cup cooked	0.16	15	12
Green beans	1 cup cooked	0.14	13	11
Cheddar cheese	1 ounce	0.11	10	8
Spinach	1 cup cooked	0.10	9	8
Strawberries	1 cup fresh	0.10	9	8
Chicken breast	½ breast roasted	0.10	9	8
Sole/flounder	3 ounces baked	0.07	6	5
Orange	1 medium fresh	0.06	5	5
Bread, whole wheat	1 slice	0.05	5	4
Bean sprouts	1 cup stir-fried	0.04	4	3
Cantaloupe	1 cup fresh	0.03	3	2
Apple	1 medium fresh	0.02	2	2

*Dietary Reference Intake

FIGURE 10.2   **Check Your Diet for Vitamin B₂ (Riboflavin)**

Using all of the foods and portion sizes in Table 10.2, "check" your daily diet in the following way:

1. Give yourself 5 (√) for each serving you eat in a day if the food provides less than 100%–80% of the DRI.
2. Give yourself 4 (√) for each serving you eat in a day if the food provides 79%–50% of the DRI.
3. Give yourself 3 (√) for each serving you eat in a day if the food provides 49%–25% of the DRI.
4. Give yourself 2 (√) for each serving you eat in a day if the food provides 24%–10% of the DRI.
5. Give yourself 1 (√) for each serving you eat in a day if the food provides 10% of the DRI.
6. No (√) for foods providing less than 10% of the DRI.

SCORE	15 or more (√)	Congratulations! Your riboflavin intake is more than adequate. Keep up the good work.
	14–10 (√)	You're doing fine. Relax and continue eating a well-balanced diet.
	9–5 (√)	You're getting about 50%–100% of the DRI for this vitamin.
	4–0 (√)	You could use a little help in getting enough of this vitamin. Refer to "great diet ideas" in this section.

well founded. Suddenly, consumers were clamoring for the return of paper cartons to replace the ubiquitous plastic gallon jugs.

The opaque jugs do allow a certain amount of light to pass through, but riboflavin loss is less compared to milk in glass bottles. Many consumers recall the days when the milk delivery man left glass milk bottles on the front doorstep in the morning. This should have accounted for riboflavin deficiency en masse for Americans, but this was not the case. While cartons are preferable, consumers who buy plastic gallons can minimize losses by returning the milk jug to the refrigerator as soon as possible. Those who prefer plastic can take comfort in riboflavin's availability from so many sources in the American diet. Studies have shown that the small loss from plastic jugs probably doesn't adversely affect most people's diets.

Recently, riboflavin made a bit of news when a study on migraine headaches hit the newsstands. Earlier, researchers had theorized that problems in energy metabolism may play a role in the development of migraines, and limited studies suggested that high-dose riboflavin was effective in preventing migraines. The authors of the recent study compared a 400 mg dose of riboflavin and placebo for three months in fifty-five migraine patients.

> **FOUR-STAR FOODS**
>
> Brewer's yeast
> Yogurt
> Mushrooms
> Ricotta cheese

Riboflavin supplementation beat the placebo in reducing the frequency of migraine attacks, with 59 percent of patients reporting improvement. No serious side effects of the supplement occurred. The researchers concluded that because of its "high efficacy, excellent tolerability, and low cost, riboflavin is an interesting option for migraine prevention." They suggested that more studies be done to compare riboflavin supplements to current drug treatments for migraine.

Vitamin B₃ (Niacin)

The disease pellagra had been known for centuries to be associated with diets using corn as the staple food, but the exact cause remained illusive. The first mention of pellagra was by the Spanish physician Casals in 1735. He described a dread disease that would go on to claim countless victims around the world among corn-eating populations for the next 200 years.

In the early 1900s, as pellagra continued to baffle scientists, it reached epidemic proportions in the southern United States. Scientists believed it was caused by an infectious agent or some toxin in corn until an American researcher, Goldberger, figured out that pellagra was caused by a still-unknown nutrient deficiency. A study in 1937 showed that nicotinic acid cured pellagra in dogs, and within a year doctors began using the compound to cure the disease in people.

Pellagra produces symptoms known as the three Ds: dementia, diarrhea, and dermatitis. Usually the final D, death, was the result. It's not surprising that early scientists couldn't figure out the corn connection. Although corn contains a fair amount of niacin, a protein in corn binds niacin, making it unavailable for absorption in the intestine. Soaking the corn in an alkaline solution releases the niacin, making it available for absorption.

This is the reason why Hispanic populations never were affected by pellagra, since they traditionally soak corn in lime water before making tortillas. But when Spanish explorers brought corn back to Europe from the New World, they weren't aware of the importance of the soaking step. This is what led to widespread niacin deficiency in Europe.

The term *niacin* is a generic name for two compounds, nicotinic acid and nicotinamide or niacinamide. Niacin functions as part of two important coenzymes that together help over 200 enzymes that depend on the vitamin to carry out chemical reactions. These coenzymes are contained in every cell of the body and are present whenever energy is released from chemical reactions. In addition, niacin is important in helping to make new compounds, especially those containing fat.

The U.S. diet provides more than adequate amounts of niacin. Good sources include whole grain or enriched grain products and meats (see Table 10.3 and Fig. 10.3). The units of measure are niacin equivalents (NE) which take into account the body's ability to convert the amino acid tryptophan into niacin. One NE, which is 1 mg of niacin, is equivalent to 60 mg of tryptophan. Surveys showed that most Americans had little difficulty meeting the 1989 RDA, and the new DRI is lower at 16 NE for men and 14 NE for women. However, some special groups who may be vulnerable include people who abuse alcohol and those who are poorly nourished. Pellagra is still a problem in Asia and Africa.

One of the most interesting facts about niacin is its cholesterol-lowering effect. Large doses of niacin (3,000 mg/day) had been shown in several studies to significantly lower blood cholesterol. One such study treated thirty-one subjects with 4 mg of nicotinic acid daily for six weeks in a highly controlled research environment, known as a metabolic ward. In all subjects, total cholesterol was significantly reduced, including the artery-clogging fractions, LDL and VLDL, which is a precursor to LDL. An added bonus was an increase in HDL. This helpful cholesterol carrier is notorious for the limited means by which it can be effectively raised.

The common side effect of large doses, anywhere from 3 to 9 grams a day, is an uncomfortable flushing of the skin, called "niacin flush," which is caused by the dilation of blood vessels. This could be more than just an annoying problem for people with asthma or ulcers. In several studies of niacin's cholesterol-lowering effect, subjects dropped out because of this side effect. A recent study in forty-two men and women suggests that an aspirin regimen of 325 mg/day is effective in preventing this pesky reaction. Other studies indicate that only the nicotinic acid form causes the skin reaction, not the nicotinamide form. Another way to prevent side effects is to use a slow-release capsule.

GREAT DIET IDEAS

1. Fish such as tuna, salmon, and halibut are excellent sources of niacin and offer an alternative to red meat at mealtimes.

2. Mushrooms are a very low-calorie, high-niacin food. One cup provides approximately 50 percent of the DRI. Try them fresh, in soups and salads, or in a stir-fry.

3. Meats are a great source of niacin. However, vegetarians can ensure adequate intake by consuming other high-niacin foods including peanuts, brewer's yeast, potatoes, dried peach halves, asparagus, cantaloupe, kidney beans, broccoli, and squash.

TABLE 10.3   **Where to Find Vitamin B₃ (Niacin)**

Food	Portion Size	Niacin (mg)	% of DRI* Women	% of DRI* Men
Chicken breast	¼ roasted skinless	11.8	84	74
Tuna, in water	3 ounces canned	11.3	81	71
Beef liver	3.5 ounces braised	10.7	76	67
Brewer's yeast	1 ounce	10.7	76	67
Salmon	3 ounces broiled	8.6	61	54
Mushrooms	1 cup cooked	7.0	50	44
Halibut	3 ounces broiled	6.1	44	38
Peach halves	10 dried	5.7	41	36
Pink salmon	3 ounces canned	5.6	40	35
Pork chop	3.5 ounces roasted	5.5	39	34
Lamb chop	3.5 ounces braised	5.5	39	34
Turkey	3.5 ounces skinless	5.4	39	34
Sirloin steak	3.5 ounces broiled	4.3	31	27
Ground beef	3.5 ounces lean baked	4.2	30	26
Peanuts	1 ounce dried unsalted	4.0	29	25
Baked potato	1 whole	3.3	24	21
Sole/flounder	3 ounces baked	2.5	18	16
Kidney beans	1 cup canned	2.4	17	15
Braunschweiger	1 ounce, tube type	2.3	16	14
Shrimp	3 ounces boiled	2.2	16	14
Wheat bran	¼ cup	2.0	14	13
Asparagus	1 cup cooked	2.0	14	13
Oysters	3 ounces raw	1.7	12	11
Sardines	2 sardines in oil	1.3	9	8
Crabmeat	3 ounces canned	1.2	9	8
Bread, whole wheat	1 slice	1.0	8	6
Summer squash	1 cup cooked	1.0	8	6
Cantaloupe	1 cup fresh	0.9	6	6
Peach	1 fresh medium	0.9	6	6
Spinach	1 cup cooked	0.9	6	6
Broccoli	1 cup cooked	0.8	6	5
Green beans	1 cup cooked	0.6	4	4
Milk, 2%	8 ounces	0.2	1	1
Apple	1 fresh medium	0.1	<1	<1
Cheddar cheese	1 ounce	0	0	0

*Dietary Reference Intake

FIGURE 10.3   **Check Your Diet for Vitamin B$_3$ (Niacin)**

Using all of the foods and portion sizes in Table 10.3, "check" your daily diet in the following way:

1. Give yourself 5 (√) for each serving you eat in a day if the food provides less than 100%–80% of the DRI.
2. Give yourself 4 (√) for each serving you eat in a day if the food provides 79%–50% of the DRI.
3. Give yourself 3 (√) for each serving you eat in a day if the food provides 49%–25% of the DRI.
4. Give yourself 2 (√) for each serving you eat in a day if the food provides 24%–10% of the DRI.
5. Give yourself 1 (√) for each serving you eat in a day if the food provides 10% of the DRI.
6. No (√) for foods providing less than 10% of the DRI.

SCORE	15 or more (√)	Congratulations! Your niacin intake is more than adequate. Keep up the good work.
	14–10 (√)	You're doing fine. Relax and continue eating a well-balanced diet.
	9–5 (√)	You're getting about 50%–100% of the DRI for this vitamin.
	4–0 (√)	You could use a little help in getting enough of this vitamin. Refer to "great diet ideas" in this section.

An even more recent study supported a beneficial effect on HDL cholesterol. One hundred patients with heart disease and high cholesterol or low HDL started the study with a niacin supplement of 100 to 250 mg twice daily. They gradually increased the dose to 1,000 mg twice a day over four to eight weeks. The doses were split to minimize side effects. The group had a 13 percent reduction in total cholesterol, a 31 percent increase in HDL, and a 32 percent decrease in the cholesterol-to-HDL ratio, a simple but effective calculation of heart attack risk.

A subgroup of thirty-nine patients taking less than 1,000 mg per day had only a 5 percent reduction in total cholesterol, but still enjoyed a 29 percent increase in HDL and a 24 percent decrease in the cholesterol-to-HDL ratio. About a third of the patients reported side effects, and four decided to drop out because of them. The results were impressive, even in the lower-dose group, since low HDL may be more predictive of heart attack than an elevated total cholesterol. The authors concluded that niacin is an effective and inexpensive treatment in improving the cholesterol-to-HDL ratio; splitting the dose cuts down on side effects.

> **FOUR-STAR FOODS**
> _____
> Chicken breast
> Tuna
> Beef liver
> Brewer's yeast

What about safety? Some researchers have cited other potential side effects besides the relatively innocuous skin tingling, including liver damage and stomach ulcers at extremely high doses. Some people using a high dose to lower cholesterol have also reported gastrointestinal side effects such as indigestion, nausea and vomiting, and diarrhea. But the potential for liver damage is by far the most serious side effect. Experts estimate that serious side effects probably only occur at doses of 2,000 to 6,000 mg. The potential benefit of niacin supplements in lowering cholesterol may warrant using it, but only under the supervision of a physician.

RESEARCH UPDATE ON NIACIN

Heart Disease: Niacin's effects on cholesterol may not be the only protection against heart disease. A Swedish study reported that the nutrient has other positive effects on blood that may prevent heart attacks. The study included twenty-three men with high blood triglycerides, a risk for heart disease, and patients received 4,000 mg of niacin for six weeks. Researchers found that the niacin treatment had the expected effect on blood lipids: It

(Continued)

reduced triglycerides, LDL, and VLDL, and raised HDL. They also found that the level of fibrinogen, needed for clotting which precedes a heart attack, was significantly reduced by the niacin supplement. Their conclusion was that treatment with niacin not only improves blood lipid problems but also affects other aspects of blood which can help protect against heart attack.

The HDL Effect: The authors of this study stated that niacin is the most potent agent for increasing plasma HDL, and they were interested in knowing how the vitamin works. Using niacin-treated cells, in an in vitro study, they found that niacin selectively lowers the liver's removal of HDL without affecting the liver's removal of other cholesterol particles. The net effect is that cholesterol is removed from circulation more efficiently, a process known as reverse cholesterol transport.

Absorption of Minerals: The researchers of this study noted that niacin is able to form complexes with essential trace metals and wanted to know if the vitamin exerts a beneficial effect on absorption of those minerals. Using human red blood cells, their results suggest that niacin may play an important role in enhancing the body's ability to use two key minerals, zinc and iron.

Chapter Eleven

Vitamins B$_6$ (Pyridoxine), B$_{12}$ (Cyanocobalamin), and Folic Acid

Vitamin B$_6$

Vitamin B$_6$ has created a stir within the past few years. Most recently, the focus has been on some groups of Americans who may need more of the vitamin than the rest of us. Other hot issues have been the use of B$_6$ in the treatment of premenstrual syndrome (PMS) and carpal tunnel syndrome. While these issues seem timely, this B vitamin has suffered relative obscurity since its discovery in 1934.

The scientist who first identified vitamin B$_6$ reported that it was "that part of the vitamin B complex which cures a dermatitis developed by rats," and in fact dubbed it "the rat antidermatitis factor." How's that for humble beginnings? More than ten years later, researchers realized that there were several forms of the "rat antidermatitis factor" and curing itchy skin on a rat was the least of the new vitamin's abilities.

Three forms of the vitamin exist: pyridoxine (PN), pyridoxal (PL), and pyridoxamine (PM), which are relatives because of their chemical structure and some of their functions. PN is the major form of the vitamin in plant foods, while the other two forms are present in animal foods. All these forms are converted by the liver, red blood cells, and a few other tissues to the main active form, pyridoxal phosphate (PLP), which we'll call B_6.

One important role of vitamin B_6 is as a coenzyme in chemical reactions related to protein metabolism. The liver is able to swap the nitrogen-containing amine group on one amino acid to another, called the transaminase reaction. This reaction makes it possible for the liver to produce new amino acids that it needs, so that you don't have to ensure you eat foods containing all twenty-one amino acids. Only nine are essential and must come from the diet. The liver utilizes the rest as the building blocks for new proteins. The body's cells are constantly making new proteins, protein for replacing old cells and tissues and for making enzymes.

One example of the kinds of reactions B_6 helps with is the conversion of the amino acid tryptophan to the B vitamin niacin and

> ## GREAT DIET IDEAS
>
> 1. A baked potato provides 54 percent of the DRI for vitamin B_6. Try one for lunch with fat-free sour cream or fat-free salad dressing.
> 2. Have a banana with corn flakes for breakfast. This supplies about 90 percent of the DRI for vitamin B_6.
> 3. Try poaching, grilling, or broiling salmon for a quick meal.
> 4. A meal of 3 ounces of trout, 1 cup of spinach, and a baked potato provides 123 percent of the DRI for vitamin B_6.
> 5. For vegetarians, five servings of fruits and vegetables per day can provide adequate amounts of vitamin B_6 if they include bananas, spinach, watermelon, soybeans, cantaloupe, avocados, cauliflower, broccoli, potatoes, and asparagus.

the neurotransmitter serotonin. Serotonin is important in sleep and a general feeling of well-being. Because of its function in making serotonin and other neurotransmitters, researchers have learned that B$_6$ is crucial to the development of the nervous system. Other interesting reactions that depend on B$_6$ include the production of a part of hemoglobin, the protein that carries oxygen in the blood, and lecithin, which makes up cell membranes. The vitamin also helps out in producing new glucose to maintain blood glucose within a normal range, making this energy source available to all cells.

The last decade has witnessed a virtual explosion of B$_6$ research, yielding exciting new roles for it. Studies have shown that the vitamin is involved in cognitive development, immune function, and the activation of certain hormones. A more controversial area has been a possible role for B$_6$ in cholesterol metabolism, with early studies showing that the vitamin either lowered cholesterol or kept it from rising. Although it's not

> ### FOUR-STAR FOODS
> Beef liver
> Baked potato
> Salmon
> Banana

clear if the relationship is direct, higher blood levels of the vitamin are linked to higher HDL and lower LDL cholesterol, at least in monkeys. Vitamin B$_6$ does appear to play a role in lowering another risk factor for heart disease, homocysteine, probably along with other B vitamins.

The Right Amount

The new DRI significantly changed the 1989 RDA in several ways. The amount for adults was reduced to 1.3 mg for men and women, but an age category was added with a different recommendation. The DRI for men over the age of fifty is 1.7 mg, and for women it is 1.5 mg. The best sources include chicken, fish, kidney, liver, pork, and eggs, each containing about .4 mg in a 3-ounce serving (see

Table 11.1 and Fig. 11.1). Legumes and some grains are fair sources, but dairy products and red meats are low in B$_6$. Although you can find B$_6$ in a variety of foods, several factors can increase requirements for the nutrient. Processing can destroy up to 70 percent of the vitamin during freezing, milling, and other common manufacturing practices.

Many prescription drugs interfere with B$_6$ metabolism, and oral contraceptives head the list. However, while contraceptives lower plasma levels of PLP, scientists aren't sure if this increases the risk for deficiency. Another drug that can pose problems is INH, which is used to treat tuberculosis. The drug has a structure similar to that of B$_6$ and takes its place at sites where the vitamin exerts its effects, but it doesn't do the vitamin's job. This is a common source of B$_6$ deficiency. Alcohol is probably more of a concern because it actually destroys B$_6$. When the body metabolizes alcohol, the first step forms acetaldehyde, a toxic compound. Acetaldehyde pries B$_6$ from its place on enzymes, causing it to break down and be excreted.

For quite some time, researchers had believed that B$_6$ deficiency was uncommon, probably occurring along with other B vitamin deficiencies in malnourished people. But some nutrition researchers aren't so sure. They cite the growing list of factors that can interfere with B$_6$ or affect how the body uses the vitamin. The first question is, what happens to people who are deficient?

Because of B$_6$'s functions in protein metabolism, deficiency should cause severe effects in this area, and because of the vitamin's role in tryptophan conversion, you might expect niacin status to be in jeopardy. Certainly, as protein intake increases, the need for B$_6$ increases, and only people whose diets are low in niacin would suffer any effects in status of that vitamin if B$_6$ intake is off. More current thinking suggests that, instead of overt problems, the effects of suboptimal B$_6$ status may be more subtle. The first deficiency symptoms could describe any number of modern people: irritability, insomnia, and weakness. Eventually, the situation gets worse with problems in nerve function, weakened immune defenses, and even convulsions.

TABLE 11.1 **Where to Find Vitamin B$_6$ (Pyridoxine)**

Food	Portion Size	B$_6$ (mg)	% of DRI*
Beef liver	3.5 ounces braised	0.91	70
Baked potato	1 whole	0.70	54
Salmon	3 ounces cooked	0.70	54
Banana	1 peeled	0.66	51
Chicken breast	½ breast skinless	0.51	39
Corn flakes	1 cup	0.50	38
Avocado	½ average	0.48	37
Trout	3 ounces broiled	0.46	35
Turkey	3.5 ounces skinless	0.46	35
Brewer's yeast	1 ounce	0.45	35
Sirloin steak	3.5 ounces broiled	0.45	35
Pork chop	3.5 ounces roasted	0.45	35
Spinach	1 cup cooked	0.44	34
Soybeans	1 cup cooked	0.40	31
Wheat germ	¼ cup	0.38	29
Tuna, in water	3 ounces canned	0.30	23
Navy beans	1 cup cooked	0.30	23
Sunflower seeds	¼ cup dry	0.30	23
Turnip greens	1 cup cooked	0.26	20
Cauliflower	1 cup cooked	0.26	20
Broccoli	1 cup cooked	0.24	18
Green pepper	1 whole	0.24	18
Watermelon	1 cup fresh	0.23	18
Ground beef	3.5 ounces lean baked	0.22	17
Asparagus	1 cup cooked	0.22	17
Figs	5 dried	0.21	16
Cantaloupe	1 cup fresh	0.18	14
Sole/flounder	3 ounces cooked	0.18	14
Mustard greens	1 cup cooked	0.16	12
Zucchini	1 cup cooked	0.14	11
Milk, 2%	8 ounces	0.11	8
Orange	1 fresh medium	0.10	8

(*Continued*)

TABLE 11.1 **(Continued)**

Food	Portion size	B₆ (mg)	% of DRI*
Green beans	1 cup cooked	0.10	8
Apple	1 fresh medium	0.07	5
Bread, whole wheat	1 slice	0.05	4

*Dietary Reference Intake for men and women ages 19–50 years.

FIGURE 11.1 **Check Your Diet for Vitamin B₆ (Pyridoxine)**

Using all of the foods and portion sizes in Table 11.1, "check" your daily diet in the following way:

1. Give yourself 5 (√) for each serving you eat in a day if the food provides less than 100%–80% of the DRI.
2. Give yourself 4 (√) for each serving you eat in a day if the food provides 79%–50% of the DRI.
3. Give yourself 3 (√) for each serving you eat in a day if the food provides 49%–25% of the DRI.
4. Give yourself 2 (√) for each serving you eat in a day if the food provides 24%–10% of the DRI.
5. Give yourself 1 (√) for each serving you eat in a day if the food provides 10% of the DRI.
6. No (√) for foods providing less than 10% of the DRI.

SCORE	15 or more (√)	Congratulations! Your B₆ intake is more than adequate. Keep up the good work.
	14–10 (√)	You're doing fine. Relax and continue eating a well-balanced diet.
	9–5 (√)	You're getting about 50%–100% of the DRI for this vitamin.
	4–0 (√)	You could use a little help in getting enough of this vitamin. Refer to "great diet ideas" in this section.

One of the first group researchers pointed to as being at high risk for B₆ deficiency were the elderly; studies showed many older people had low levels of the vitamin in various body tissues. Soon after, others countered that the depressed levels were merely reflecting natural changes of aging, not necessarily inadequate vitamin status. The consensus now suggests that the elderly probably do have a higher requirement for the vitamin as a result of age-related changes in B$_6$ metabolism. Most nutritionists expected to see a higher B$_6$ recommendation for the elderly with the new DRI, and technically the committee did this by creating a new age category. But since the previous RDA was higher, the net effect is actually a reduction in the vitamin recommendation.

Another vulnerable group appears to be Americans who smoke, based on several studies reporting that smoking increases the requirement for B$_6$. One study compared levels of B$_6$ compounds in smokers, ex-smokers, and nonsmokers and found that blood levels of the vitamin were significantly lower in smokers than in ex-smokers and nonsmokers. The only problem was that when researchers measured vitamin levels inside red blood cells, they found no differences among the three groups. Since B$_6$ does its coenzyme dance inside of cells, they questioned the significance of low blood levels. One important finding was that B$_6$ blood levels may not be the best, and are certainly not the only indicator of B$_6$ status.

Too Much?

When the RDA Committee last updated this vitamin's recommendation, it stated that acute toxicity of the vitamin is low. But a spate of studies proposing B$_6$ as an effective treatment for PMS and carpal tunnel syndrome in which high doses were used seemed to suggest otherwise. Some women who took daily doses of 2,000 mg or more over a six-month period for PMS, which is 125 times the RDA, reportedly developed numbness and other nerve problems. However, they all recovered completely within six months after stopping the supplement. Other studies that purportedly showed the same nerve problems at lower doses, even as low as 100 mg, were not well controlled, and women took the vitamin for almost three years. A recent review of vitamin toxicity suggests that most of the concerns are exaggerated, but it's the length of time a supplement is used rather than the amount that predicts nerve problems.

RESEARCH UPDATE: B_6

Carpal Tunnel Syndrome: Carpal tunnel syndrome (CTS) is becoming a problem in many industries as more workers are using computers and other machines requiring repetitive movement, so the growing interest of environmental engineers is not a surprise. Researchers in Oregon measured blood levels of B_6 and vitamin C in 441 adults from six industries and a university exercise study to evaluate if the vitamin was related to either CTS symptoms or slowing, an effect short of CTS but indicating beginning nerve function problems. Men who didn't use vitamin supplements and had lower B_6 levels reported more pain, tingling, and waking up in the night. In this same group, the ratio of vitamin C to B_6 blood levels was directly associated with the occurrence of the symptoms. The authors concluded that there is an important interaction between vitamin C and B_6 related to outright symptoms of CTS and deficits in nerve function.

Premenstrual Syndrome: Australian researchers examined the rates of PMS symptoms in 310 women aged eighteen to forty-five, studying treatments used and the perceived effectiveness of treatments. They found that between 11 and 32 percent of women reported severe changes during the premenstrual phase of the cycle on ten symptoms typically used to assess PMS, with the highest rates for changes in mood. Eighty-five percent of women reported trying treatments for PMS, and many reported having tried multiple treatments. The most common treatments included painkillers, rest, increased fluid intake, and exercise. Almost 33 percent of the women had used these treatments or combinations of them. The women reported that the three most effective treatments were dietary changes, evening primrose oil, vitamins (including B_6), and exercise. Half the women had sought help from their doctors, and 45 percent said they'd like help in fighting PMS. The exact role of B_6 isn't clear, but it appears that especially in women who may have suboptimal intakes of the vitamin, supplements and other treatments may be helpful.

Heart Disease: Scientists have proven that high blood levels of homocysteine (HC) is a risk factor for cardiovascular disease (CVD), and more studies are showing that HC levels are related to levels of folate and vitamin B$_6$. European researchers recently evaluated the relationship between HC, B vitamins, and CVD. They studied 750 patients with diagnosed CVD and 800 control subjects matched for age and sex. They checked blood levels of HC, folate, B$_6$, and B$_{12}$ in red blood cells. The results showed that HC levels were associated with a higher risk for CVD independent of all other risk factors, such as high blood cholesterol and high blood pressure. In a boost for two of the B vitamin trio, red blood cell levels with the lowest levels of B$_6$ and folate were associated with a higher risk even in the control subjects; this risk was also independent of known risk factors. Interestingly, folate's protective role had to do with lowering HC levels, but B$_6$'s benefit was independent of HC level. The authors concluded that lower blood levels of folate and vitamin B$_6$ increase risk for CVD, and that clinical trials will help evaluate the effectiveness of treatment with these vitamins in both those with existing CVD and healthy people.

Dutch researchers followed up with clinical trials in 89 patients with CVD and 277 healthy controls. They assessed the effects of supplementation with the B vitamin trio using 5 mg folic acid, 0.4 mg B$_{12}$, and 50 mg B$_6$. Vitamin supplementation normalized HC levels in 87 percent of subjects, compared to 23 percent in the placebo group. Even in subjects with previously normal HC levels, multivitamin supplementation significantly lowered HC levels. In the group with normal HC, folate by itself lowered HC as well as the combination of B vitamins. By itself, B$_{12}$ supplementation lowered HC only slightly, by about 10 percent. The researchers concluded that the trio was effective in lowering HC levels in both CVD patients and healthy subjects, but even supplementation with 0.5 mg of folic acid alone led to a significant reduction in blood HC levels.

Epilepsy: Chinese researchers evaluated the effectiveness of B$_6$ to treat seizures in infants and young children. Of ninety infants and children with recurrent convulsions due to acute infections, they treated forty with a high dose of B$_6$; fifty subjects served as the controls. They also gave all subjects antiepileptic drugs, and they measured effectiveness by the number of convulsions per day and

(Continued)

the duration of individual seizures. The results showed that treatment effectiveness for the B_6 group and control group was 92.5 percent and 64 percent, respectively. They also found no adverse effects of vitamin supplementation. The authors concluded that B_6 is a safe, effective, and inexpensive adjunct to routine treatment of recurrent seizures in children.

Infections: This French study examined vitamin C and B_6 status, two vitamins playing a role in immune function in elderly people. The researchers wanted to know if infections could alter the metabolism of either of these vitamins in patients over the age of seventy-five. They divided the patients into three groups: eight with acute infections, four who were malnourished, and six healthy controls. They assessed vitamin status four times for twenty-one days and found significant differences in vitamin levels among the various groups: B_6 levels were higher in the control group than either the infection or malnourished groups, and vitamin C levels were lower in the infection group compared to the malnourished and control groups. The researchers concluded that their study suggests that acute conditions such as infection may influence vitamin B_6 and C metabolism. However, results from more studies are needed to see if supplementation of these two important vitamins is called for during infection.

Kidney Disease: Kidney disease causes problems involving several nutrients, and a recent study from Europe investigated whether B_6 supplements could be helpful in patients who need kidney dialysis. Kidney disease affects B_6 for several reasons. The drug furosemide, which doctors commonly use to help the body excrete extra water and minerals, causes increased urinary excretion of the vitamin in people with chronic renal failure. Another problem is the dialysis procedure itself, especially the type of dialysis which uses the patient's abdominal membrane as the filter. A drug treatment used by kidney patients to be able to make new red blood cells, erythropoietin, also appears to adversely affect B_6. While B_6 normally gets used up in the making of red blood cells, this process is accelerated with erythropoietin treatment in patients using hemodialysis, the other type of dialysis, in which a machine filters the blood. Hemodialysis patients had improvement in immune function when taking daily B$_6$ supplements of 50 mg. To prevent B$_6$ deficiency, the authors recommended a daily 5 mg supplement in dialysis patients not taking erythropoietin and 20 mg for those who do.

Nausea in Pregnancy: Nausea and vomiting during pregnancy are common, but when severe they threaten a woman's nutritional status and increase the risk for poor outcomes. In an effort to find effective treatments, alternative therapy researchers reviewed recent American and international studies. They found several studies which considered the effects of acupressure, ginger, and B$_6$ on nausea and vomiting of pregnancy. After analyzing these studies, they reported beneficial effects were found for all three of these interventions, although the evidence for acupressure yielded mixed results. They stated that "there is a dearth of research to support the efficacy of common remedies for nausea and vomiting of pregnancy." And they concluded that the "best-studied alternative remedy" is acupressure, which may help some women, and evidence suggests that ginger and vitamin B$_6$ may also be beneficial.

Another concern was the possibility that B$_6$ supplements could cause kidney stones, but studies showing this effect had used a special form of the vitamin, not the standard form. A subsequent study actually reported that men who took more than 40 mg a day had a lower risk for kidney stones than those consuming less than 3 mg.

Besides PMS, people have used B$_6$ to treat carpal tunnel syndrome. People with carpal tunnel syndrome suffer from numbness and tingling pain, which starts in the hand and wrist and radiates up the arm, sometimes causing swelling. There is some evidence to suggest that one possible cause in some people is B$_6$ deficiency. This may be especially true in older adults, in whom clinicians have identified a B$_6$-responsive carpal tunnel syndrome.

Pyridoxine is one of the B vitamins that has piqued the interest of researchers relative to a number of human conditions and diseases. While the results of some of their efforts remain to be proven, there is good evidence for several of these hypotheses. Is B_6 an effective treatment for PMS and carpal tunnel syndrome? Look at the latest studies in the "Research Update" and decide for yourself.

Recommendation Too Low?

Most people in the United States eat too much protein, many consuming up to three times the RDA. As protein intake increases, the requirement for B_6 also rises. Researchers at Washington State studied B_6 requirements in young women eating a high-protein diet of .71 g/pound of body weight, which is almost double the RDA and varied the B_6 content of the diet. The diet was lacto-ovovegetarian (no meats but including dairy products and eggs). Over the course of a month on the various diets, the researchers evaluated the women's B_6 status every week. They found that the amount of dietary B_6 the women needed to maintain the vitamin's functions was 1.94 mg, or 20 percent above the 1989 RDA, which was in effect when the researchers carried out the study. Interestingly, most studies show that men tend to eat even more protein than women, and diets containing meat products are more likely to be higher in protein than vegetarian diets such as the one used in this study. The authors concluded that since most Americans eat almost twice the amount of protein set by the RDA, the 1989 RDA for B_6 wasn't adequate. The study was done before the new DRI, which lowered the recommendation for this vitamin.

Vitamin B_{12} (Cyanocobalamin)

The long history of Vitamin B_{12}'s discovery is strewn with wrong turns, mysterious clues, frustration, and finally scientific heroes who saved thousands of people from an agonizing and ghastly death—a "pernicious" death. Today, this B vitamin is a familiar friend: you may have heard of friends or relatives going to their doctors' offices for B_{12} injections for a purported energy boost. No one is quite sure why these friends and relatives receive the injections, and they aren't sure either. But there's nothing mysterious about the crucial role this B vitamin plays in human health, not the least of which is to prevent pernicious anemia, the deficiency disease.

The search for B$_{12}$ led scientists on a not-so-merry chase that began in 1822 when a Scottish doctor reported on the "history of a case of anemia." The name they eventually gave this anemia was on target, considering the devastating neurologic damage it causes. The Scottish doctor felt that the disease was the result of a digestion or absorption problem; he just didn't know what. After his report, scientists began to study pernicious anemia with some vigor, and it was an American doctor who deduced the nutrition connection forty years later.

In between these clues, another B vitamin threw researchers off the scent by causing an anemia resembling pernicious anemia. A deficiency of the B vitamin folate causes a macrocytic anemia in which red blood cells are much larger than normal, similar to pernicious anemia. A breakthrough occurred when researcher Wills reported on a macrocytic anemia in pregnant Hindu women from Bombay. Her team of workers successfully treated the women with a yeast extract and later reproduced what they thought was the same anemia in monkeys. They cured the monkeys' anemia with a crude liver extract and named its magic ingredient "the Wills Factor." They found that when they purified the crude extract, it could still cure the monkeys, who actually had B$_{12}$ deficiency, but not the women, who had a folate deficiency. Although Wills and her team couldn't quite put the last pieces in the puzzle, their work paved the way for the next two sleuths of science.

In 1926, Minot and Murphy tied up some loose ends and developed an oral liver therapy which proved to be an effective treatment for pernicious anemia, work for which they later won the Nobel Prize. The vitamin yielded its secrets in the late 1940s when two independent groups isolated it in crystalline form, and the tangle between folate and B$_{12}$ began to make sense.

It's not surprising that B_{12}'s discovery was long and arduous. This vitamin has the most complex chemical structure of all the vitamins. If you need any more proof of B_{12}'s complicated nature after reading about its history, just think about this—it took more than 100 scientists in nineteen countries spanning a decade to understand it! Its chemical name, cyanocobalamin, arises from the presence of the mineral cobalt in the vitamin, and it has a characteristic deep red hue. Interestingly, the other part of its name comes from cyanide used in the synthetic process, not the naturally occurring form.

To understand B_{12}'s role in the body, you have to factor in folate or folic acid. It's not surprising that those earlier researchers and physicians got them mixed up for so many years, because the vitamins are tightly entwined in the body's metabolism. The vitamins team up to make DNA in the following way: B_{12} acts as a coenzyme with an inactive form of folate to help convert one amino acid into another. In the process, folate becomes activated so that it's able to participate in DNA synthesis. Without B_{12}, folate remains inactive and unable to do its job. It's biggest task is DNA synthesis so folate deficiency brings this process to a crawl, and one of the consequences is that new red blood cells aren't able to divide and mature. The anemia shows up as those large and immature red blood cells. It's in this way that a B_{12} deficiency causes a lack of folate.

This explains the similarity in symptoms of B_{12} and folate deficiency. It also explains why folate had not been available as a single vitamin supplement until recently. If a person has B_{12} deficiency, taking a folate supplement will make the red blood cells normal again, lulling the person or their doctor into thinking the problem is resolved. But folate only masks the symptoms of B_{12} deficiency, and the disease continues to ravage the nervous system until the damage is irreversible and soon causes death.

B_{12} also does some important things on its own. One important function is to maintain the sheath that surrounds nerve fibers and promotes their growth. This role in nerve function accounts for the neurologic damage when there is a deficiency. B_{12} also appears to play a role in the activity of bone cells and their metabolism. The studies mentioned for B_6 also included a role for B_{12} in lowering homocysteine levels and reducing the risk for heart disease.

How the Body Absorbs B_{12}

The absorption of B_{12} is almost as complicated as its history, chemical structure, and relationship with folate. When you eat food that contains the vitamin, acid and digestive enzymes made by the stomach free it from other compounds. Once loose, a compound made by the stomach called the R-binding protein snatches it up. Meanwhile, another compound the stomach makes, the intrinsic factor, watches this new couple with envy like a secret admirer, wanting a dance with B_{12} but having to wait its turn. The intrinsic factor is actually B_{12}'s soul mate, but doesn't get its chance until the couple reaches the small intestine. In the last few inches of the small intestine, with the end of the dance seconds away, intrinsic factor makes its move, and R-protein backs off. Intrinsic factor claims his prize and escorts the alluring vitamin into the absorbing cells of the small intestine—oh yes, they do live happily ever after.

But the ending isn't always so happy, because some people who have stomach or intestinal problems may not be able to absorb B_{12}. The stomach plays a key role in B_{12} absorption by making acid, R-protein, and intrinsic factor. Since it's the acid that keeps the R-protein and B_{12} together in the stomach, people who've had stomach surgery to reduce acid production, most commonly for ulcers, may have a problem. Some people have a condition known as achlorhydria in which the stomach cells don't produce enough acid. This often happens to the elderly, probably due to aging, and chronic gastritis can also cause low acid production. Besides acid, stomach problems or surgery can affect the organ's ability to make both R-protein or intrinsic factor.

Even after clearing the stomach, the small intestine has to be in tip-top shape to do its part in B_{12} absorption. In the neutral environment of the small intestine, the R-protein lets go and the intrinsic factor complex with B_{12} is favored. This new complex moves along to the terminal ileum, the last part of the small intestine, where absorption of the vitamin occurs. Problems affecting the terminal ileum, such as Crohn's and celiac disease, will reduce B_{12} absorption and often cause the deficiency. Since absorption of the vitamin depends on intrinsic factor and the digestive tract for all the steps, a B_{12} supplement has to be given by injection into the muscle.

FOUR-STAR FOODS

Clams
Beef liver
Oysters
Clam chowder

People who've had portions of the small intestine removed, especially the terminal ileum, may develop B_{12} deficiency. Another intestinal problem known as blind loop syndrome can cause deficiency. Blind loop develops when a portion of the small intestine is bypassed, either intentionally as in surgery or from inflammation, causing bacteria to grow. The bacteria need B_{12}, too, so they use it up before the person gets a chance to absorb it.

Where Is B_{12}?

The new DRI raised the recommendation for the vitamin from 2 micrograms to 2.4. They also inserted a warning phrase: "10 to 30 percent of older adults malabsorb the vitamin, so these people need to insure the recommended level from foods or supplements." The targets are achievable for people who don't have an absorption problem and who eat animal products. A little further down the food chain, bacteria, fungi, and algae can make their own B_{12}, but yeasts, plants, animals, and humans have to consume sources of the vitamin. Animal products are the main sources of B_{12} (see Table 11.2 and Fig. 11.2), and the bacteria living in your intestine add a bit, too. Plants don't naturally contain B_{12}, but they may become contaminated with microorganisms who make the vitamin, leaving some behind for the animal or person to eat. Sometimes food labels can be a bit misleading when they show plant products containing B_{12}; if it is present, it's in an inactive form the body can't use. However, some plant products, such as soy milk, have vitamins added during processing, which make them a good source for strict vegetarians. The wide availability of the vitamin makes overt deficiency due to poor dietary intake uncommon, with deficiency arising from absorption problems a more likely cause. Some studies show that strict vegetarians who don't eat any animal products, not even dairy foods, may have low blood levels of B_{12} and are at risk for a deficiency.

Research into the B_{12} status of elderly Americans is of current interest. One recent study from the Netherlands reported that blood levels of B_{12} were low in 6 percent of healthy elderly and 5 percent of elderly people in hospitals. And researchers have found high levels of the vitamin's metabolites, which accumulate when vitamin status is impaired, in 63 percent of healthy and 82 percent of hospitalized elderly. This led the authors to conclude that many elderly people are at risk for B_{12} deficiency and that measurement of the vitamin's metabolites is a more sensitive indicator that could help in early detection of deficiency. Of special concern was a study from 1988 which reported that the elderly may have psychiatric symptoms of

---

GREAT DIET IDEAS

1. A breakfast of ¾ cup raisin bran with 8 ounces of low-fat milk provides 120 percent of the DRI for vitamin B_{12}.
2. Try low-fat cottage cheese with fruit as a snack.
3. A 3-ounce portion of salmon, tuna, or rabbit provides 100 percent of the DRI for vitamin B_{12}.
4. Oysters and clams are excellent sources of B_{12}. They can be served steamed or in stews and chowders.
5. Some great meat-free sources of vitamin B_{12} are vegetarian burgers, raisin bran, miso, tempeh, cottage cheese, milk, buttermilk, and yogurt.

B_{12} deficiency from nerve damage even before anemia develops. And a recent study from Scotland supports results from earlier studies by showing that the elderly often have low blood levels; tests for B_{12} status shouldn't be limited to looking for large red blood cells, or macrocytic anemia.

TABLE 11.2   **Where to Find Vitamin B_{12} (Cyanocobalamin)**

Food	Portion Size	Vitamin B_{12} (mcg)	% of DRI*
Clams	3 ounces cooked	84.1	3,500
Beef liver	3.5 ounces braised	71.0	3,000
Oysters	3 ounces cooked	32.5	1,350
Clam chowder	1 cup	10.3	427
Rabbit	3.5 ounces roasted	8.3	346
Braunschweiger	1 ounce, tube type	5.2	216
Sirloin steak	3.5 ounces broiled	2.9	119
Salmon	3 ounces cooked	2.7	113
Tuna, in water	3 ounces canned	2.5	106
Lamb chop	3.5 ounces braised	2.3	95
Vegetarian burger	½ cup	2.0	83
Raisin bran	¾ cup	2.0	83
Ground beef	3.5 ounces lean baked	1.7	71
Cottage cheese, 1% fat	1 cup	1.4	58
Sole/flounder	3 ounces cooked	1.3	54
Shrimp	3 ounces cooked	1.3	54
Halibut	3 ounces broiled	1.2	50
Milk, 2%	8 ounces	0.89	37
Frankfurter, beef	2 ounces	0.88	37
Ham	3.5 ounces cooked	0.74	29
Tempeh	½ cup	0.70	29
Pork chop	3.5 ounces roasted	0.60	25
Buttermilk, cultured	8 ounces	0.54	23

TABLE 11.2 (Continued)

Egg	1 whole fresh	0.50	21
Turkey	3.5 ounces skinless	0.37	15
Canadian bacon	2 slices cooked	0.36	15
Miso	½ cup	0.29	12
Chicken breast	½ breast, skinless	0.29	12
Yogurt, low fat	8 ounces	0.24	10
Cheddar cheese	1 ounce	0.23	10
Goat's milk	8 ounces	0.16	7
Baked potato	1 whole	0	0
Bread, whole wheat	1 slice	0	0
Apple	1 fresh medium	0	0
Spinach	1 cup cooked	0	0

*Dietary Reference Intake

FIGURE 11.2 Check Your Diet for Vitamin B$_{12}$ (Cyanocobalamin)

Using all of the foods and portion sizes in Table 11.2, "check" your daily diet in the following way:

1. Give yourself 5 (√) for each serving you eat in a day if the food provides less than 100%–80% of the DRI.
2. Give yourself 4 (√) for each serving you eat in a day if the food provides 79%–50% of the DRI.
3. Give yourself 3 (√) for each serving you eat in a day if the food provides 49%–25% of the DRI.
4. Give yourself 2 (√) for each serving you eat in a day if the food provides 24%–10% of the DRI.
5. Give yourself 1 (√) for each serving you eat in a day if the food provides 10% of the DRI.
6. No (√) for foods providing less than 10% of the DRI.

SCORE	15 or more (√)	Congratulations! Your B$_{12}$ intake is more than adequate. Keep up the good work.
	14–10 (√)	You're doing fine. Relax and continue eating a well-balanced diet.
	9–5 (√)	You're getting about 50%–100% of the DRI for this vitamin.
	4–0 (√)	You could use a little help in getting enough of this vitamin. Refer to "great diet ideas" in this section.

RESEARCH UPDATE: B_{12} DEFICIENCY

Researchers reported on a case study of a fourteen-year-old boy who developed severe anemia from B_{12} deficiency at the onset of puberty. The researchers believe that he had the deficiency for almost ten years. When they asked what he usually ate, they found that his intake consisted of mainly chips, ice cream, fruit, and cola. His only source of the B vitamin was from the ice cream and small amounts from occasional slices of chicken meat. After doctors diagnosed his deficiency, they prescribed a more normal diet and he rapidly improved. Although the case study only gives information on one person, it demonstrates that B_{12} deficiency from improper food intake can and does occur.

Folic Acid (Folate)

Folic acid has been garnering its share of attention in the past few years, and the future portends more of the same if current research is any indication. The two main areas of interest include the vitamin's protective roles against a devastating birth defect and heart disease. The former has captured the attention of women and the food industry because of newly passed legislation, while the link to heart disease prevention is continually being strengthened.

Although folate and B_{12} work together, folate has a life of its own. It also has a tongue-twisting name, pteroylglutamic acid, which isn't much of an improvement over some of the first stabs at naming it: vitamin M, vitamin B_{10}, vitamin B_{11}, rhizopterin, and factor SLR. The friendlier name they settled on, folate, indicates that they first isolated it from spinach and figured out that leafy greens were good sources. After haggling over the name, scientists started realizing how important the vitamin is to the body. Through its role in DNA and RNA synthesis, folate helps in the production of many important compounds, including amino acids and cell parts. It's also involved in the metabolism of fat.

After you eat foods that contain folate, intestinal enzymes have to pull off chemical groups called glutamates before the intestine can absorb the vitamin. Some compounds in foods, especially in yeast and legumes, can interfere with the enzymes and reduce absorption. Although any part of the small intestine can absorb folate, the preferred site is the first third of the small intestine. Similar to other nutrients, a variety of intestinal diseases that affect the absorbing cells of the small intestine can cause a folate deficiency, especially in the upper part of the intestine.

Various drugs, such as those used to control epilepsy, can also cause problems with folate absorption. Chronic alcohol abuse often causes folate deficiency for several reasons, one of which is the liver's role in activating folate, as well as alcohol's interference with the intestinal enzymes. Any factor that increases the metabolic rate, such as infection or trauma, will increase the need for folate.

Where's the Folate?

A variety of foods contain folate, and good sources include liver, leafy vegetables, legumes, and whole grains (see Table 11.3 and Fig. 11.3). Although folate occurs in many foods, one difficulty in getting enough folate is that the vitamin is extremely sensitive to heat and other processing methods. Some studies show that up to 95 percent of the folate can be lost by long cooking times and commercial processes such as canning. This may be the reason that surveys show some Americans aren't getting enough of the vitamin, with one recent study reporting that 88 percent of Americans don't meet the RDA.

The National Institute of Medicine recently revised the 1989 RDA in switching to the new DRI and increased the recommended level of folate by twice the amount to 400 micrograms. Interestingly, the 1989 RDA committee had cut the folic acid RDA by half, from the previous level of 400 micrograms! The Institute of Medicine broke new ground and suggested that Americans either take supplements or eat foods that are fortified with the vitamin. Fortified sources include most breakfast cereals and other grain products. Their rationale was based on two facts: dietary surveys show that Americans don't eat enough foods high in folate, and new studies show that the body absorbs twice as much folate in the synthetic form as from the natural form of folate in foods. Food manufacturers use the synthetic form when they fortify food products.

TABLE 11.3   **Where to Find Folate**

Food	Portion Size	Folate (mcg)	% of DRI*
Pinto beans	1 cup cooked	294	74
Asparagus	1 cup cooked	264	66
Spinach	1 cup cooked	262	66
Navy beans	1 cup cooked	255	64
Beef liver	3.5 ounces braised	217	54
Black-eyed peas	1 cup cooked	209	52
Great northern beans	1 cup cooked	181	45
Turnip greens	1 cup cooked	170	43
Lima beans	1 cup cooked	156	39
Kidney beans	1 cup canned	129	32
Broccoli	1 cup cooked	104	26
Corn flakes	1 cup	100	25
Parsley	1 cup chopped	92	23
Beets	1 cup cooked	90	23
Wheat germ	¼ cup	82	21
Romaine lettuce	1 cup chopped	76	19
Cauliflower	1 cup cooked	64	16
Pineapple juice	8 ounces canned	58	15
Orange	1 fresh medium	47	12
Zucchini	1 cup cooked	30	8
Peanuts	1 ounce dried	29	7
Cantaloupe	1 cup fresh	27	7
Winter squash	1 cup cooked	26	7

TABLE 11.3 (Continued)

Strawberries	1 cup fresh	26	7
Grapefruit juice	1 cup canned	26	7
Egg	1 whole fresh	23	6
Green beans	1 cup cooked	22	6
Tofu	½ cup raw	19	5
Tomato	1 whole raw	18	5
Bread, whole wheat	1 slice	14	4
Bean sprouts	1 cup fresh	12	3
Milk, 2%	8 ounces	12	3
Sirloin steak	3.5 ounces broiled	10	3
Cheddar cheese	1 ounce	5	1
Apple	1 fresh medium	4	1

*Dietary Reference Intake

FIGURE 11.3   Check Your Diet for Folate

Using all of the foods and portion sizes in Table 11.3, "check" your daily diet in the following way:

1. Give yourself 5 (√) for each serving you eat in a day if the food provides less than 100%–80% of the DRI.
2. Give yourself 4 (√) for each serving you eat in a day if the food provides 79%–50% of the DRI.
3. Give yourself 3 (√) for each serving you eat in a day if the food provides 49%–25% of the DRI.
4. Give yourself 2 (√) for each serving you eat in a day if the food provides 24%–10% of the DRI.
5. Give yourself 1 (√) for each serving you eat in a day if the food provides 10% of the DRI.
6. No (√) for foods providing less than 10% of the DRI.

SCORE   15 or more (√)   Congratulations! Your folate intake is more than adequate. Keep up the good work.

14–10 (√)   You're doing fine. Relax and continue eating a well-balanced diet.

9–5 (√)   You're getting about 50%–100% of the DRI for this vitamin.

4–0 (√)   You could use a little help in getting enough of this vitamin. Refer to "great diet ideas" in this section.

Another important reason for the huge increase in the recommended folate level is the evidence for protection against neural tube defects (NTDs) in newborns. The neural tube is tissue which gives rise to the embryo's brain and spinal cord. Defects of this tube, of which spina bifida is the most common, cause profound disabilities and high risk for infant death. In a recent survey targeting the concern for NTDs, the Centers for Disease Control and Prevention (CDC) reported that only 32 percent of women of childbearing age take folic acid supplements.

Women Need More Folate

Evidence for folic acid's role in preventing NTDs had continued to mount in the late 1980s. Initially, experts thought that women needed to ensure an adequate intake only during pregnancy. But later studies began to suggest that it was actually a woman's prepregnancy folic acid status that was key to the development of NTDs in her newborn. By 1992, the U.S. Public Health Service recommended that all women of childbearing age consume 400 micrograms of folate daily to reduce their risk for bearing a child with NTDs. The agency had projected that of the nearly 4,000 annual cases of the disease, half could be prevented by adequate folic acid intake.

FOUR-STAR FOODS

Pinto beans
Asparagus
Spinach
Navy beans

In response, the Food and Drug Administration (FDA) issued a proposal and three final rules in March 1996. These included a requirement for folic acid fortification of many enriched grain products and authorization for specific health claims. A food item meeting the FDA criteria for "good source" can make the health claim regarding NTDs. One constraint is that a food item containing folate and also 100 percent of the RDA for vitamins A and D cannot use the health claim because of A and D's adverse effects on fetal health.

By January 1998, the requirement for folic acid fortification of enriched grain products took effect. All commercial grain products have to be enriched with between 430 micrograms and 1,400 micrograms per pound. Breakfast cereals may contain up to a daily dose of folic acid. Examples of the types of grain products covered by the requirement include flour, self-rising flour, corn grits, cornmeal, farina, rice, macaroni products, noodles, breads, rolls, and buns. The FDA is concerned about some people getting too much folate because of food fortification. The existing food additive regulation wouldn't have been able to prevent excessive intakes because it permitted the addition of folic acid to virtually any food, so the FDA amended the regulation.

> ## Great Diet Ideas
>
> 1. Use dry beans in soups or as a main-dish salad.
> 2. Use fresh spinach in salads and lasagna, or serve cooked with fresh lemon juice.
> 3. Make a fresh salad with spinach, romaine, tomatoes, broccoli, cauliflower, and beets.
> 4. A meal of 3.5 ounces of beef liver, 1 cup of asparagus, and 1 cup of lima beans provides 159 percent of the DRI of folate.
> 5. A breakfast of 1 cup of cornflakes in milk with a fruit salad of 1 cup cantaloupe, strawberries, and orange provides 54 percent of folate needs for the day.

What About Men?

The folate focus had been almost exclusively on women, until some intriguing studies began to link the vitamin with heart disease. The evidence that folate lowers homocysteine, and therefore heart disease risk (CHD), is strong—strong enough that experts are now reminding men that they need folate, too. Early work on the relationship between CHD and homocysteine suggested that three B vitamins were helpful in reducing blood levels of this risk factor, but it wasn't clear which of the trio was responsible. In 1995, researchers at the University of Washington reported on their meta-analysis of thirty-eight CHD and folic acid studies. Based on their analysis, they projected that increasing the American intake of the vitamin could prevent 56,000 CHD deaths annually.

More evidence on folic acid's protection against CHD came recently from a study at the Cancer Bureau in Ottawa, Ontario. Canadian researchers examined blood levels of folic acid collected from over 5,000 people in 1970. The prospective study showed that subjects with the lowest blood levels of the vitamin were 69 percent more likely to die of CHD in subsequent years. But remember the caveat from Chapter 1 about the strength of a research study: even if epidemiologic studies show a link, it may not be causal. The proof of the connection can only come from an intervention or clinical trial.

Proof came fast! Within the span of six months, a spate of converging studies crowned folate as the unequivocal champ in the fight against CHD, relegating its B brethren to the stage wings. The most recent of these studies came from the Dutch researchers mentioned in the B_{12} section which supported the homocysteine-lowering effect of the three Bs, but also showed that folate could go it alone.

Other studies included a study from Ireland in which researchers gave thirty healthy men varying doses of folate for six weeks, checking homocysteine levels throughout. Folate effectively lowered homocysteine in all groups except the group with already low levels of the risky compound. They found that 200 micrograms was the most effective dose, compared to 100 and 400 micrograms. This was good news, since there is less concern for toxicity when the supplement is a lower dose but still effective.

With the recent legislation mandating food fortification and consumers taking supplements to get the vitamin's purported protective effects, the FDA's concern about people getting too much folate is shared by others. In a review of vitamin toxicity, one expert put the concern in perspective. His review stated that the three main concerns regarding folate safety are masking pernicious anemia, interference with zinc function, and interference with certain medications.

As for the first, studies show that only doses exceeding 5,000 micrograms can mask the anemia, and those studies used injections, not oral supplements. The second concern for zinc is more problematic. Folate does seem to interfere with the body's use of this important mineral, based on lab studies. But the proof again has to come from intervention studies, and large clinical trials using the recommended 400 microgram or slightly higher dose through pregnancy don't show problems with zinc. Furthermore, the reviewer points to the large body of evidence showing "clear benefit in reducing risk of NTDs."

As for folate's interference with certain medications, two drugs are of concern—an antiepilepsy drug, diphenylhydantoin, and a chemotherapy drug, methotrexate. The review concludes that studies show that folate can reduce diphenylhydantoin's effectiveness in controlling seizures, but the doses used were from 5,000 to 30,000 micrograms. Interestingly, for methotrexate, recent studies show that a 1,000 microgram folate supplement actually reduced the drug's toxic effects without reducing its overall effectiveness.

RESEARCH UPDATE: FOLATE

Depression: A recent review suggests that there is good evidence from clinical reports of depressed patients and lab studies to suggest a role for folate in neuropsychiatric disorders. Lab studies have given scientists enhanced understanding of the role of folate in brain function, and it appears that symptoms of depression are the most common neuropsychiatric problem of folate deficiency. Researchers point to studies showing either borderline low or

(Continued)

deficient blood levels of folate levels in up to 38 percent of people diagnosed with depressive disorders. Folate's part in depression may be related to the neurotransmitter serotonin. Scientists believe that folate supplements, and compounds related to the vitamin, may be useful in the near future in treating depressed patients.

Folate Status of Adolescent Girls: Canadian researchers were interested to know if there was an association between dietary fiber intake and the folate status of adolescents girls and the rate of vitamin deficiency in this group. They tested the girls for blood levels of folate and asked questions about dietary habits. Of the girls who practiced lactoovovegetarianism, 14 percent had low folate intakes, and 26 percent of girls who ate all foods had diets low in folate. In this last group, 23 percent had low blood levels of folate, indicating deficiency. Even with the large number of girls with folate deficiency, they had normal homocysteine levels. The researchers found that a higher intake of fiber was associated with higher blood levels of folate, which made sense considering that some of the best sources are fruits and vegetables. But the authors said that the fiber probably promoted bacterial synthesis of the vitamin in the intestine. They suggested that recommendations to increase fiber intake might be helpful in improving folate status.

Diabetes and Heart Disease: Researchers in Sweden had reported that people with diabetes had high levels of homocysteine, which they believed was one of the reasons for the increased risk for and early development of heart disease.

In a more recent study, they analyzed homocysteine blood levels and two vitamins known to lower it, folate and B_{12}, in fifty patients with insulin-dependent diabetes. The results showed that diabetic patients who developed the disease at the youngest ages and who had difficulty controlling their diabetes were those most prone to rapid increases in homocysteine. They also found that in this group of patients, the high homocysteine was probably also due to low levels of folate.

Blood Vessels: A study from the Netherlands may provide evidence for another role of folate in protecting against heart attacks. Scientists have known for a while that when the activity of nitric oxide (NO) in the body is abnormal, it may lead to the development of cardiovascular disease (CVD). The NO compound is protective, so that low levels of NO may pose a risk for CVD. One of folate's relatives plays a critical role in the production of NO, so the researchers wanted to test the theory that folate supplementation could restore NO activity in people with genetically high blood cholesterol. They studied the effects of folate supplements on ten patients with high blood cholesterol and ten control subjects. They found that folate improved blood vessel dilation problems in the treatment group but didn't affect the controls. Folate didn't have a direct effect on NO production, but it did reduce levels of free radicals. The authors concluded that the folic acid supplement restored proper blood vessel functioning in patients with genetic high blood cholesterol, probably by reducing the breakdown of NO.

Chapter *Twelve*

Pantothenic Acid, Biotin, and Choline

Pantothenic Acid

Although pantothenic acid isn't exactly a newcomer to the vitamin scene, having been isolated in 1938, most people have never heard of this B vitamin. You can probably blame its anonymity on the fact that scientists had identified it and were able to synthesize it long before they knew its role in human nutrition. It wasn't until the late 1940s that researchers began to unravel the mystery, and part of the work earned one of them a Nobel Prize. Its name is derived from the Greek word *pant*, meaning everywhere, in recognition of its wide distribution in nature.

The main function of this vitamin is as a component of an important coenzyme which is vital for over 100 chemical reactions. Some of these include the release of energy from carbohydrates and the synthesis of fats, hormones, and hemoglobin. It's

FOUR-STAR FOODS
Beef liver
Mushrooms
Avocado
Salmon

also involved in nerve transmission by its role in making neuro-transmitters.

Scientists haven't found too many cases of pantothenic acid deficiency in humans, but they have seen enough ill effects in lab animals, such as growth retardation, infertility, and sudden death, to know it is essential. They suspect that pantothenic acid deficiency is responsible for a condition called "burning feet syndrome" reported in prisoners of war and malnourished people in the Far East. It appears that although it's rare, pantothenic acid deficiency probably causes general failure of all the body's systems.

The vitamin is widely distributed in foods, in virtually all animal foods and plant products such as grains and legumes (see Table 12.1 and Fig. 12.1). The 1989 RDA didn't include a full-fledged recommendation for pantothenic acid because of a lack of sufficient evidence. But in the new DRI this is set at 5 mg for adults. It seems to be easy for the intestine to absorb pantothenic acid from foods, and a limited amount travels to the liver and kidney for storage.

Some interesting human studies have shown that high doses promoted faster wound healing after surgery, and in animals pantothenic acid seems to accelerate the normal healing process. Scientists think pantothenic acid works in these stressful situations

GREAT DIET IDEAS

1. Since pantothenic acid is found in many different foods, a balanced diet should provide the recommended daily intake.
2. Try avocado sliced on a salad or in a dip such as guacamole.
3. A meal of 3 ounces of salmon, 1 baked potato, 1 cup of broccoli, and 8 ounces of milk provides 75 percent of the recommended daily intake for pantothenic acid.
4. Try soups and dishes that contain lentils, split peas, and mushrooms.
5. Try a main-dish salad with chicken breast, spinach, mushrooms, broccoli, and avocado.

TABLE 12.1   Where to Find Pantothenic Acid

Food	Portion Size	Pantothenic Acid (mcg)	% of DRI*
Beef liver	3.5 ounces braised	4.6	91
Mushrooms	½ cup boiled	1.7	34
Avocado	1 medium	1.7	34
Salmon	3 ounces cooked	1.4	28
Lentils	1 cup boiled	1.3	25
Split peas	1 cup boiled	1.2	23
Potato	1 whole baked	1.1	22
Turkey	3.5 ounces skinless	0.94	19
Pomegranate	1 medium raw	0.92	18
Chicken breast	½ roasted skinless	0.83	17
Peanuts	1 ounce dried	0.79	16
Milk, 2%	8 ounces	0.78	16
Sweet potato	1 whole baked	0.74	15
Chickpeas	1 cup canned	0.72	14
Wheat germ	¼ cup	0.66	13
Pork chop	3.5 ounces roasted	0.65	13
Egg	1 whole fresh	0.63	13
Broccoli	1 cup cooked	0.50	10
Ham	3.5 ounces cooked	0.47	9
Sole/flounder	3 ounces cooked	0.43	9
Kidney beans	1 cup canned	0.38	8
Sirloin steak	3.5 ounces broiled	0.37	7
Corn	1 cup boiled	0.36	7
Orange	1 fresh medium	0.35	7
Watermelon	1 cup fresh	0.34	7
Ground beef, lean	3.5 ounces baked	0.27	5
Spinach	1 cup cooked	0.26	5
Bread, whole wheat	1 slice	0.18	4

(Continued)

TABLE 12.1   (Continued)

Food	Portion Size	Pantothenic Acid (mcg)	% of DRI*
Tuna, in water	3 ounces canned	0.18	4
Macaroni, enriched	1 cup cooked	0.16	3
Cheddar cheese	1 ounce	0.12	2
Green beans	1 cup cooked	0.12	2
Apple	1 fresh medium	0.08	1
Corn flakes	1 cup	0.05	1
Margarine	1 teaspoon, tub type	0	0

*Dietary Reference Intake

FIGURE 12.1   **Check Your Diet for Pantothenic Acid**

Using all of the foods and portion sizes in Table 12.1, "check" your diet in the following way:

1. Give yourself 5 (√) for each serving you eat in a day if the food provides less than 100%–80% of the DRI.
2. Give yourself 4 (√) for each serving you eat in a day if the food provides 79%–50% of the DRI.
3. Give yourself 3 (√) for each serving you eat in a day if the food provides 49%–25% of the DRI.
4. Give yourself 2 (√) for each serving you eat in a day if the food provides 24%–10% of the DRI.
5. Give yourself 1 (√) for each serving you eat in a day if the food provides 10% of the DRI.
6. No (√) for foods providing less than 10% of the DRI.

SCORE	15 or more (√)	Congratulations! Your pantothenic acid intake is more than adequate. Keep up the good work.
	14–10 (√)	You're doing fine. Relax and continue eating a well-balanced diet.
	9–5 (√)	You're getting about 50%–100% of the DRI for this vitamin.
	4–0 (√)	You could use a little help in getting enough of this vitamin. Refer to "great diet ideas" in this section.

by its effect on the adrenal glands, which produce stress hormones such as adrenalin. Recent studies suggest that this vitamin is non-toxic, with doses of 10 grams producing no ill effects, although a few studies have reported gastrointestinal symptoms at high doses.

Biotin

Biotin is another B vitamin with which most people aren't familiar, even though its discovery dates back to the 1930s. The nutrient plays an important role as a coenzyme in several metabolic reactions. One such reaction is crucial in the pathway that releases energy from carbohydrate. Other reactions include making new glucose and fatty acids, and the breakdown of amino acids.

Biotin is another B vitamin that you can find in a wide variety of foods, although the amounts are limited. Good sources include liver, egg yolks, whole grain cereals, soy flour, and yeast (see Table 12.2 and Fig. 12.2). One interesting interaction occurs with raw eggs, which contain the protein avidin. Avidin grabs the biotin, also present in the egg,

> ### GREAT DIET IDEAS
>
> 1. Use granola as a cereal, or a snack, or mix it into yogurt and puddings.
> 2. Try wheat germ in casseroles and breads, or on cereal.
> 3. Use Ry-Krisp with peanut butter and jelly for snacks.
> 4. For lunch, try egg noodles with fat-free Italian dressing mixed with vegetables.
> 5. In moderation, eggs can be part of a healthy diet. Try them scrambled, poached, or hard boiled.

and prevents the intestine from absorbing it. Cooking the egg causes the proteins to uncoil and not work as they should, and, in the case of avidin, it's just as well. In virtually all the documented deficiency cases, eating raw eggs was the reason for the problem. As long as you don't eat two dozen raw eggs every day, the amount experts say produces the deficiency, you don't have much to worry about.

Scientists had known that intestinal bacteria produce the vitamin, making it available to humans. However, they now believe that this is not a significant source of the vitamin. The new DRI for biotin is 30 micrograms for both men and women, and surveys show that Americans consume 28 to 42 micrograms per day of this nutrient. The vitamin is relatively nontoxic, with doses as high as 60 mg for six months causing no ill effects.

FOUR-STAR FOODS

Eggs
Wheat germ
Ry-Krisp
Granola

Researchers were the first to see biotin deficiency in humans when they fed volunteers a biotin-deficient diet in the 1940s. Within five weeks of the deficient diet, all volunteers had changes in mental status, nausea and anorexia, and numbness and tingling. In two more weeks, they developed dermatitis on their arms and legs. Biotin injections reversed all the symptoms. If the deficiency had been allowed to progress, however, the volunteers would have lost their hair and suffered from weakened immunity. Infants may be born with a genetic defect, organic acidemia, that produces biotin deficiency. Without receiving biotin injections, the infants would soon die.

Choline

Before the recent DRI update, this nutrient was relegated to the lists of also-rans or, worse, vitamin impostors. But the Institute of Medicine recently raised this nutrient from obscurity to a more legitimate status. Soon after scientists discovered choline in 1862, they were able to synthesize the compound. And as researchers began to learn about choline's key functions, the only question that remained was, is choline an essential nutrient? At first glance, most scientists said an emphatic no, since the body can make choline out

TABLE 12.2   **Where to Find Biotin**

Food	Portion Size	Biotin (mcg)	% of DRI*
Egg	1 whole fresh	10.0	33
Wheat germ	¼ cup toasted	7.0	23
Ry-Krisp	½ ounce	6.8	23
Granola	¼ cup w/raisins	5.0	17
Egg noodles	1 cup cooked	4.0	13
Almonds	1 ounce whole natural	1.0	3
Pistachios	1 ounce	1.0	3
Corn meal, yellow	1 ounce	1.0	3
Macaroni, enriched	1 cup cooked	0	0
Corn flakes	1 cup	0	0

*Dietary Reference Intake

FIGURE 12.2   **Check Your Diet for Biotin**

Using all of the foods and portion sizes in Table 12.2, "check" your daily diet in the following way:

1. Give yourself 5 (√) for each serving you eat in a day if the food provides less than 100%–80% of the DRI.
2. Give yourself 4 (√) for each serving you eat in a day if the food provides 79%–50% of the DRI.
3. Give yourself 3 (√) for each serving you eat in a day if the food provides 49%–25% of the DRI.
4. Give yourself 2 (√) for each serving you eat in a day if the food provides 24%–10% of the DRI.
5. Give yourself 1 (√) for each serving you eat in a day if the food provides 10% of the DRI.
6. No (√) for foods providing less than 10% of the DRI.

(*Continued*)

FIGURE 12.2   **(Continued)**

SCORE	15 or more (√)	Congratulations! Your biotin intake is more than adequate. Keep up the good work.
	14–10 (√)	You're doing fine. Relax and continue eating a well-balanced diet.
	9–5 (√)	You're getting about 50%–100% of the DRI for this vitamin.
	4–0 (√)	You could use a little help in getting enough of this vitamin. Refer to "great diet ideas" in this section.

of several compounds. As that is the test for essentiality, the consensus ran in favor of the nays for several years.

Those researchers who believed choline to be essential cited these facts: human cells grown outside the body require choline to survive; people fed a choline-deficient diet have low blood levels of the nutrient; malnourished patients have low blood levels of choline; and in other primates, a choline-deficient diet causes liver failure. But other scientists countered that just because a person's blood level is low doesn't mean the nutrient is essential. A quick look at some of choline's roles would suggest an important compound that may deserve to be called essential. Some of these roles include helping to make phospholipids such as lecithin and the neurotransmitter acetylcholine.

FOUR-STAR FOODS

Beef liver
Cauliflower
Peanuts
Peanut butter

What finally won over the committee with the power to confer the honor of essentiality or at least conditional essentiality? Probably studies showing that in periods of human growth and development, the need for choline outpaces the amount the body can make. This suggests that, at least during critical periods, a person needs to have a dietary source of choline. Other conditions that call for more choline than the body can produce include aging and certain neurologic disorders. Some research has suggested that choline may be a protective factor in several chronic diseases, but the work is mostly theory based on lab studies.

Foods containing choline include eggs, liver and other organ meats, milk, legumes, and nuts (see Table 12.3 and Fig. 12.3). People who take lecithin as a dietary supplement add to their choline intake. One problem can be our intestinal bacteria; they often add to our nutrient status as with vitamin K, but they tend to break down choline, making it unavailable for the body to absorb. The DRI committee set an Adequate Intake (AI) for this newcomer of 550 micrograms for men and 425 micrograms for women.

You might recall from Chapter 1 that an AI is different from an RDA in that for many nutrients (choline is one) the research data aren't quite as solid as for other nutrients. Both an AI and an RDA are estimates of how much of a particular nutrient you need, but when scientists have better evidence, they set

GREAT DIET IDEAS

1. A meal of 3.5 ounces of beef liver, 1 cup of cauliflower, 1 baked potato, 8 ounces of grape juice, and a banana provides 176 percent of the DRI for choline.

2. Adding a leaf of iceberg lettuce to a sandwich provides 10–15 percent of daily choline needs.

3. Instead of cola, try mixing 8 ounces of grape juice with 12 ounces of ginger ale for a "choline cocktail." It provides approximately 25 percent of the DRI for choline.

4. A snack of 1 ounce of peanuts and 8 ounces of milk provides about 30 percent of the DRI for choline.

5. Try a peanut butter and jelly sandwich with 8 ounces of grape juice for lunch and get nearly 50 percent of the DRI for choline.

an RDA. The DRI committee also set a tolerable upper limit (UL) for choline of 3.5 mg, stating that doses above this level could cause low blood pressure or a fishy body odor in some people.

TABLE 12.3   **Where to Find Choline**

Food	Portion Size	Choline (mcg)	% of DRI* Women	% of DRI* Men
Beef liver	3.5 ounces	583.1	137	106
Cauliflower	1 cup cooked	162.0	38	29
Peanuts	1 ounce dried	127.3	30	23
Peanut butter	2 tablespoons	124.6	29	23
Grape juice	8 ounces canned	120.0	28	22
Potato	1 whole baked	103.2	24	19
Iceberg lettuce	1 leaf raw	58.6	14	11
Tomato	1 whole raw	52.9	12	10
Milk, whole	8 ounces	36.6	9	7
Orange	1 fresh medium	28.0	7	5
Banana	1 whole peeled	27.4	6	5
Bread, whole wheat	1 slice	24.2	6	4
Cucumber	½ cup raw	11.3	3	2
Beef steak	3.5 ounces	7.5	2	1
Apple	1 fresh medium	3.7	<1	<1
Egg	1 fresh whole	2.1	<1	<1
Ginger ale	12 ounces	0.73	<1	<1
Butter	1 teaspoon	0.21	<1	<1
Margarine	1 teaspoon, tub type	0.15	<1	<1
Corn oil	1 tablespoon	0.04	<1	<1

*Dietary Reference Intake

FIGURE 12.3   Check Your Diet for Choline

Using all of the foods and portion sizes in Table 12.3, "check" your daily diet in the following way:

1. Give yourself 5 (√) for each serving you eat in a day if the food provides less than 100%–80% of the DRI.
2. Give yourself 4 (√) for each serving you eat in a day if the food provides 79%–50% of the DRI.
3. Give yourself 3 (√) for each serving you eat in a day if the food provides 49%–25% of the DRI.
4. Give yourself 2 (√) for each serving you eat in a day if the food provides 24%–10% of the DRI.
5. Give yourself 1 (√) for each serving you eat in a day if the food provides 10% of the DRI.
6. No (√) for foods providing less than 10% of the DRI.

SCORE		
	15 or more (√)	Congratulations! Your choline intake is more than adequate. Keep up the good work.
	14–10 (√)	You're doing fine. Relax and continue eating a well-balanced diet.
	9–5 (√)	You're getting about 50%–100% of the DRI for this vitamin.
	4–0 (√)	You could use a little help in getting enough of this vitamin. Refer to "great diet ideas" in this section.

Vitamins Summary

R esearch trends in the area of vitamins continue to point to their emerging and expanding role in human health and disease prevention. The link between vitamins and health continues to excite the imaginations of both nutritionists and American consumers. And as America continues to age and more studies point to the role of vitamins in protecting against diseases such as cancer and heart disease, we'll see a continuing change in attitudes regarding the role of vitamins, moving away from the "deficiency mind-set" to a more expanded view of their place in optimal health.

Although people could theoretically get all the nutrients they need from their diets, there's a growing awareness that we may need to consider certain vitamins in a different light. Many also recognize the new social reality of our increasingly hectic lifestyle, its lightning pace making the diet more vulnerable to skipped or pared-down meals, often leaving out important vitamins.

Armed with expanding knowledge of details about vitamins such as dosage effects, absorption, and disease development, future research will help us to better understand the role of vitamins in human health and disease. With this better understanding will come bold but solid recommendations regarding optimal vitamin intakes and potential efficacy, as well as safety of supplementation. In the meantime, you may have noticed that certain foods keep showing up as good sources on almost every vitamin list.

Nutrient Powerhouses

The following foods are "nutrient powerhouses" because they are good sources of several nutrients.

Beef liver	A, K, B_2, B_3, B_6, folate, B_{12}, pantothenic acid, biotin, choline
Spinach	A, K, B_2, B_6, folate, C
Sweet potato	A, E
Milk	A, D, B_2
Potato	C, B_6, B_3, choline
Watermelon	B_1, C
Mushrooms	B_1, B_2, B_3, pantothenic acid
Broccoli	A, B_2, C, K, pantothenic acid
Sunflower seeds	B_1, B_6, E
Brewer's yeast	B_1, B_2, B_3, B_6, folate
Wheat germ	B_1, biotin
Asparagus	B_1, B_2, B_3, B_6, C, folate
Pork	B_1, B_3, B_{12}
Fortified bread/cereal	A, B_1, B_2, B_3, B_6, C, folate
Cantaloupe	A, B_3, C

A famous nutrition researcher, Alfred Harper, once pointed out that human beings are remarkably resilient and can thrive quite well on a variety of diets, proven by those diets of myriad cultures around the world. He questioned the idea that we could determine an optimum diet for every person; no one perfect diet exists. This was revolutionary thinking which remains unchallenged today, in an age where thousands of self-styled experts slug it out to impart their perfect diet plans—for a small fee, of course. Finally, do you remember the Japanese Dietary Guideline from the first chapter— the one about enjoying your meals? That advice just might be one of the wisest recommendations of all.

Glossary of Other Interesting Compounds (But Not Vitamins)

A s you probably noticed after reading the first section, the food you eat contains many other compounds that affect your health. The vitamins are only one group of nutrients among other essential ones, and a whole new category, the glamorous phytochemicals, keeps popping into your morning paper. This section is a mini-dictionary containing short descriptions of other interesting compounds, many with potential health effects, that you ran across in previous chapters. In addition, you'll find some compounds occurring in foods that aren't so friendly.

Acarbose: A naturally occurring compound which interferes with glucose absorption. It is now widely used as a drug to treat diabetes, in which it helps to prevent high blood glucose after meals. Researchers have proposed that in addition to reducing glucose absorption from the intestine, acarbose also increases the time for stomach contents to enter the intestine. Both of these effects help to prevent a large increase in blood glucose following a meal. People with both types of diabetes can use acarbose but most often will need other drugs or insulin to maintain blood glucose within normal ranges.

Acesulfame-K: An FDA-approved alternative sweetener that provides no calories and has the advantage over other alternative sweeteners of being stable when heated in cooking or baking.

Additives (food additives): Substances added to foods by manufacturers to impart some desirable characteristic such as resistance to spoilage, color, flavor, texture, stability, or nutritional value. The Food and Drug Administration (FDA), charged with regulating additives, defines them as any substances that become part of a food product when added either directly or indirectly.

Currently, the FDA estimates that about 3,000 substances are added intentionally, with another 10,000 entering food products during processing, packaging, or storage. When additives are used intentionally, the FDA says that they can be used for one or more of the following four purposes:

- to maintain or improve nutritional value
- to maintain freshness (prevent spoilage)
- to make food more appealing (taste and appearance)
- to help in processing or preparation

The categories of intentional food additives include antimicrobial agents (see *antimicrobials*), artificial colors (see *food coloring*), artificial flavors and flavor enhancers, nutrient additives, and preservatives. Surprisingly, the most common additives are sugar, salt, and corn syrup. When considered with citric acid, baking soda, vegetable colors, mustard, and pepper, they account for 98 percent by weight of all additives used in the United States. While food additives have been used for thousands of years, they continue to be a point of contention for consumers and food manufacturers. As more sophisticated technology makes possible newer processing methods, additives have kept pace. It's very likely that even more additives will become a part of our food supply.

Antimicrobials: Substances approved by the FDA for use in food products to prevent the growth of microorganisms. Antimicrobials include a wide-ranging group of additives which protect food from spoilage that results in food poisoning by inactivating microbes such as bacteria, yeasts, molds, and other fungi.

Early civilizations recognized the preservative power of two of the most commonly used antimicrobials widely in use today, salt and sugar. Salt was used thousands of years ago and continues to be used in meat and fish. Sugar is used to preserve canned and frozen fruit and in a variety of jams and jellies. Both salt and sugar function in a similar manner in food preservation by withdrawing water from the food and binding it. The microbes require water to survive and grow, and these agents deprive them of water by the binding action.

One group of antimicrobials, the nitrites, has gained notoriety by being linked to cancer-causing compounds called nitrosamines. They fulfill several functions in foods but the most important of these is to prevent the growth of a specific bacteria, clostridium botulinum, which produces the deadly toxin known as botulism. Nitrites are converted into nitrosamines in the human stomach when they combine with amines. Consider this for perspective, however—a cigarette smoker inhales 100 times more the nitrosamines than the average person gets eating bacon. Other sources of nitrosamines include beer, which provides five times the nitrosamine of bacon, and cosmetics, which deliver twice the nitrosamines of cured meat through skin absorption. Antimicrobials used include salt, sugar, nitrites, natamycin, nisin, bateriocins, potassium sorbate, and sodium propionate.

Arginine: An amino acid, not considered essential as the body can make it. It is involved in the synthesis of urea, a waste product from protein metabolism, and creatine (see *creatine*). Some studies show that this amino acid may become essential in cases of trauma, severe burns, system-wide infections, and for wound healing.

Aspartame: An alternative sweetener made from two amino acids, phenylalanine and aspartic acid. It provides calories, since it is protein, but because it's 200 times sweeter than sugar, the calories are extremely low. It breaks down when heated, so it can't be used in baking. People born with the genetic abnormality called phenylketonuria (PKU) don't have the enzyme that breaks down phenylalanine, which can accumulate and cause mental retardation. When babies are born, they're routinely tested for PKU, and, if positive, they have to avoid foods that contain phenylalanine. After the age of about ten, the diet can be less restrictive but blood levels of the amino acid must be monitored. Although some consumer groups have raised concerns about the safety of aspartame, the FDA considers the sweetener safe other than for people with PKU.

BGH (bovine growth hormone): A hormone produced by the pituitary gland of cows that stimulates growth and milk production. BGH was recently approved by the FDA for use in milk cows to increase milk production. Controversy has surrounded the commercial use of this compound for the past few years, with opponents raising potential health concerns and scientists and government officials stating that BGH is safe. Those who have raised concerns cite the increased rate of udder infection among cows treated with the hormone, which necessitates increased use of antibiotics. Antibiotics, in turn, show up in meat and milk from treated cows. Overuse of these drugs may cause microorganisms to develop resistance and spread more infectious disease. The FDA and most scientists say that this is unlikely and maintain that BGH is safe.

BHA and BHT: Preservatives used to inhibit the development of off flavors, odors, and discoloration of foods. The preservatives act as antioxidants in cereal products, baked goods, and snack foods. Studies have shown that BHT prevents cancer in animals exposed to carcinogens, and animals given BHT also live longer than controls. However, at high levels, BHT has been shown to increase cancer risk. The amount currently approved by the FDA in foods is considered safe.

Bioflavonoids (flavonoids): A group of compounds that occur naturally in plant foods, many of which have biologic activity, especially as antioxidants. When scientists first discovered the bioflavonoids, they believed the compounds to be a new vitamin, vitamin P. Researchers are interested in bioflavonoids now for their biologic activities in fighting chronic diseases such as cancer and heart disease. One of the compounds generating much interest is quercetin (see *quercetin*). Bioflavonoids are concentrated in the skin, peel, and outer layers of fruits and vegetables. Tea, coffee, and wine are also good sources of bioflavonoids.

Caffeine: A naturally occurring compound found in tea and coffee, and related to theobromine in cocoa beans (used to make chocolate). Caffeine's various and potent stimulant effects have been both praised and reviled throughout history. It stimulates the kidneys to excrete fluid and the heart to increase its work output. At varying doses, people report gastrointestinal upset, tremors, insomnia, and rapid heartbeat. At extremely high doses, over 5,000 mg, caffeine can cause convulsions, coma, and heart failure. However, at amounts provided by even excessive coffee or tea drinking, studies have not reported any long-term adverse health effects. Coffee, from an automatic drip maker, has 137 mg in a 5-ounce cup, and black tea brewed for three minutes has 42 mg in the same amount. People who need to limit or avoid caffeine include those with certain heart disorders and pregnant women, who should not exceed 2 cups a day.

Carnitine: An essential nutrient for the mealworm *Teneabrio molitor*, but not for humans. Humans can synthesize this compound under normal conditions from two amino acids, lysine and methionine, so it isn't necessary to obtain it in the diet. It now appears that some people may not synthesize an adequate amount and that some diseases can inhibit its production. Carnitine functions in fat metabolism by carrying long-chain fatty acids into the mitochondria for beta-oxidation. People who have a genetic disorder in which their bodies can't make carnitine suffer from muscle weakness, hypoglycemia, and fat accumulation between muscle fibers. To date, carnitine deficiency has been documented in premature infants maintained on IV feeding. However, low blood levels of carnitine have been noted in infants fed soy formula and in diseases which interfere with fat storage in muscle tissue. While it is a vital nutrient, supplements may not be beneficial unless you are deficient in it.

Conjugated Linoleic Acid: A group of isomers of linoleic acid, an essential fatty acid; the conjugated part of the name refers to the compounds having what chemists call conjugated double bonds. The first part of the story begins in 1987, in a research lab in the United States, when researchers discovered that an isomer (a mirror-image duplicate) of an essential nutrient appeared to possess anticarcinogenic activity. Since that initial report and several others, subsequent studies ensued linking CLA to prevention of atherosclerosis and to weight loss. The most interesting part of the story is the list of foods containing CLA, notorious for their continual appearance on nutritionists' "most not wanted" list: fried ground beef, steak, and full-fat dairy products such as cheese and ice cream.

Intriguing studies in rabbits have shown that even among those fed a high-fat diet, the addition of CLA significantly lowered LDL cholesterol without adversely affecting HDL. More impressive was the autopsy data finding that CLA–fed rabbits had less atherosclerosis. Rats fed CLA early in life also had significantly lower body fat than controls. Bodybuilders are already attempting to cash in on the muscle-promoting effects of CLA, as supplements are widely available. To date, the studies have all been laboratory investigations, either in vitro or with animals. While promising, particularly in the areas of carcinogenesis and atherosclerosis, human studies will be the true test.

Creatine: A component of creatine phosphate which acts as the body's source energy in the muscle contraction. Creatine occurs naturally in meat products. Muscle, brain, and blood all contain creatine, and small amounts are excreted into the urine. People who have severe liver disease, diabetes, or are starving, excrete high levels in the urine. It is currently of interest because of studies showing that supplements can increase athletic performance by up to 15 percent. Although that level of enhancement seems slight, to highly trained athletes who compete in various events, it can offer a competitive edge.

Cryptoxanthin: A carotenoid, of yellow pigment, that the body can convert to active vitamin A, naturally occurring in fruits and vegetables. The best sources include corn, oranges, and paprika. As with other carotenoids, researchers are studying its possible role in preventing chronic diseases.

Emulsifiers: Compounds which allow the dispersion of minute particles or globules contained in one liquid phase into another liquid phase. The typical example is of trying to mix oil and vinegar. Because vinegar is water based and oil is a lipid, combining the two liquids will result in a separation with the oil floating on the top. If an emulsifier is added, the two liquids will stay mixed. The result is salad dressing, which is a common use for emulsifiers.

These versatile compounds are also important in the baking industry. Emulsifiers improve various qualities of baked goods, including volume, uniformity, and the fineness of the grain. In preparation, dough will also handle more easily when emulsifiers are used. Some types of emulsifiers added to shortening allow a higher ratio of sugar to flour in cakes, which increases flavor without decreasing volume.

Dairy products, ice cream, and frozen desserts also benefit from the addition of emulsifiers. In frozen products, emulsifiers ensure smaller, more uniform particle size which imparts a smoother texture. Commonly used emulsifiers include glycerides (mono- and diglycerides), lecithin (see *lecithin*), polysorbate 60 and 80, and propylene glycol monostearate. In addition, some gums and starches have emulsifying properties.

Fatty Acids (FA): A group of organic acid compounds which contain the elements carbon, hydrogen, and oxygen. In nature, they usually possess an even number of carbons, anywhere from four to twenty-four, which contributes partially to their specific names. Unsaturation, also used in naming FA, refers to the number of double bonds between carbon atoms which replace hydrogen atoms. The body's inability to make a particular FA confers essentiality, which means it must be obtained from the diet.

Scientists first discovered FA and our need for them in the late 1920s and since then have studied and discussed these interesting compounds for decades. They continue to be not only intriguing and controversial to researchers, but to health-conscious consumers as well. The most recent interest relates to their possible link primarily with coronary heart disease, but also a seemingly endless list of other twentieth-century plagues.

The essential FA (EFA) are polyunsaturated (PUFA), containing more than one double bond and include linoleic, linolenic, and arachidonic acids. While arachidonic acid is considered an EFA by definition, the body can synthesize it from linoleic acid. EFAs are needed for growth, reproduction, skin maintenance, and fat utilization.

The monounsaturated fatty acids (MUFA) have one double bond, as implied by their name, and scientists have studied them since the late 1970s because of their link to heart disease. Their claim to fame was based on studies which suggested that they lowered total serum cholesterol without lowering HDL cholesterol like their PUFA counterparts do. Olive and canola oils are excellent sources of MUFA. However, food sources of saturated FA containing no double bonds, which tend to raise serum cholesterol, such as chicken, pork, and beef fat, may also contain 40 to 45 percent MUFA. Another type of FA, trans FA, produced by the commercial hydrogenation process, has been shown to adversely affect blood cholesterol levels.

Fiber: Nondigestible materials in plant products which include cellulose, hemicellulose, lignin (see *lignin*), pectins, gums, and mucilages. Humans also can't digest some fibers from animal products, including ligaments and gristle. The older term for fiber was *roughage* or *bulk*. Scientists distinguish between crude fiber and dietary fiber, relative to the procedure needed to degrade the compounds. For human health, only dietary fiber is significant. There are two main categories of fiber, soluble and insoluble, which describe the compounds' solubility in water. From a health standpoint, the difference is important.

Insoluble Fiber: These include cellulose, some hemicelluloses, and lignin. Insoluble fiber absorbs water in the colon, making the stools more bulky, which aids in elimination. This may help prevent constipation and diverticulosis. Sources of insoluble fiber include wheat bran, whole grain breads and cereals, and vegetables.

Soluble Fiber: These include gums, pectins, most hemicelluloses, and mucilages. Researchers have linked soluble fiber with reducing blood glucose in people with diabetes, lowering blood cholesterol, and preventing colon cancer. The colon cancer connection is likely related to bacteria in the colon breaking down the fiber and producing short-chain fatty acids (see *short-chain fatty acids*). Good sources include fruits, especially apples and citrus, legumes, oats, and barley.

Fish Oils: The omega FA (OFA) found primarily in fish. The omega, Greek for last, part of the name, refers to the position of the double bond starting from the first carbon from the carboxyl group end of the FA. Omega is usually followed by a number which indicates the position of the nearest double bond. Three groups of OFA which are important in the diet make up the omega-3 FA including linolenic, eicosapentaenoic (EPA), and docosahexaenoic (DHA) acids, found in fish oils. The other two EFA, linoleic and arachidonic, are examples of omega-6 FA.

Epidemiologic studies first linked omega-3 FA to low rates of heart disease among Native Alaskans who traditionally consume a high-fish diet, in particular fatty types of fish. Since then, these OFA have been studied with regard to a host of physiologic effects and disease prevention and treatment. Aside from a role in heart disease prevention, researchers have postulated that omega-3 FA may lower blood pressure, alleviate arthritic symptoms, strengthen immune function, and most recently discovered, protect kidney transplant patients from organ rejection.

It is thought that many of these possible physiologic relationships are the result of OFA's role in the biosynthesis of potent compounds known as prostaglandins, thrombaxanes, and leukotrienes, collectively termed the eicosanoids. Their physiologic effects include promoting or inhibiting the inflammatory response, platelet aggregation and adhesion, blood pressure regulation, and blood vessel constriction and dilation.

While OFA's reduction of platelet aggregation is beneficial in some people with heart disease, this effect may pose a risk in others. Some experts had theorized that hospitalized patients might be adversely affected because of prolonged bleeding time, a consequence of reduced clotting ability. However, a recent study from Harvard Medical School refutes this theory.

Food Coloring Agents: Substances approved by the FDA for use in food products to impart color. While many consumers continue to express concern about food colors, most are unaware that humans have been using coloring agents throughout history. In addition, studies have shown time and again the importance of the color of foods to humans' perception and ultimate acceptance of the food.

The practice of coloring foods appears to have begun in ancient Rome where spices such as saffron were used to both flavor and color foods. In the middle ages, Brits used coloring agents in sugar to make it rose or violet colored. And not long after, yellow color was added to butter to make it more appealing.

Regulation of colors began early in this century with congressional passage of the Food and Drug Act of 1906. Prior to this, over eighty synthetic colors were being used in foods. However, legislation approved only seven for use in foods. In addition, the act established a voluntary certification process under the aegis of the Department of Agriculture. Soon after, Congress passed the Federal Food, Drug and Cosmetic (FD&C) Act of 1938 requiring certification and transferring this function to the Food and Drug Administration (FDA).

As an additive and from a legal definition, coloring agents can consist of any dye, pigment, or other substance which adds color to food, drug, cosmetic, or even the human body itself. However, not all colors to which the FDA has given the official nod can be used in foods. Some colors are restricted to use in other products, such as cosmetics. A color which the FDA has permitted for use in foods is known as FD&C certified. The color must first pass a rigorous battery of tests performed by both the FDA and the manufacturer to ensure safety, quality, and consistency.

Some colors currently in use are exempt from the certification process as they are derived from natural sources such as vegetables. However, they must still meet FDA specifications to be approved for use. Certified colors are more commonly used by manufacturers because of greater color intensity than their natural pigment counterparts. Currently, the FDA oversees an ongoing safety review for all certified colors.

Colorant Terms: FD&C Blue No. 1, 2; Green No. 3; Red No. 3, 40; Yellow No. 5, 6 (see *tartrazine*); Citrus Red No. 2.

Exempt Colors: Annatto extract; B-Apo-8'-carotenal; beta-carotene; beet powder; caramel color; carrot oil; cochineal extract (carmine); ferrous gluconate; fruit juice; grape color extract; grape skin extract (enocianina); paprika; riboflavin; saffron; titanium dioxide; turmeric; vegetable juice.

Fructose: A sugar naturally occurring in fruits and honey, with the same chemical formula as glucose but differing in structure. It's much sweeter than table sugar, sucrose, but provides the same calories. Fructose takes longer to be absorbed into the bloodstream, and for that reason, nutritionists had thought it to be useful for people with diabetes. However, studies have shown that high levels of fructose may increase blood lipids, a problem for which people with diabetes have a high risk. In addition, high amounts of the sugar can cause diarrhea. In normal amounts, from fruits, fructose doesn't pose a problem.

Genistein: An isoflavone found in plant foods, especially soy. Current theories suggest genistein may be responsible for the protection against heart disease studies associated with eating soy foods. Some studies show that eating soy foods can reduce the risk of heart disease by 18 to 28 percent. This may be related to genistein's ability to reduce serum cholesterol levels by 3.3 percent in people with normal cholesterol levels and up to 24 percent in individuals with high cholesterol.

Genistein may reduce the risk of heart disease by preventing atherosclerosis, the deposition of plaque in the arterial wall and subsequent narrowing of the vessels. Studies suggest that it inhibits platelet aggregation and other stages of the clotting process which add to arterial injury and deposition of plaque in damaged blood vessel walls. By inhibiting the formation of plaques, genistein prevents blood vessel blockage which ultimately leads to a heart attack. Thus far, genistein's effects have been confined to the laboratory, and final confirmation awaits clinical human trials.

Genistein may also prevent breast cancer by competing with estrogen for receptor sites in breast and other tissues. By preventing estrogen from binding, genistein keeps the hormone from exerting some of its deleterious effects in these tissues. Studies have shown that genistein mimics the action of the anti-estrogen drug tamoxifen used in breast cancer therapy. Genistein also inhibits angiogenesis, the growth of new blood vessels needed to supply rapidly growing tumor cells, which may prevent benign tumors from growing. In addition, genistein inhibits tyrosine protein kinase in vitro, an enzyme produced by mutated genes that causes normal cells to become cancerous.

In contrast to breast cancer, which researchers have linked to high levels of circulating estrogen, osteoporosis may be partially the result of estrogen deficiency in postmenopausal women. Recent study of the effects of soy on bone health and heart disease found that high isoflavone treatment increased lumbar spine bone density and raised HDL and lowered LDL cholesterol.

Glutamine: A nonessential amino acid contained in a wide variety of foods. Glutamine is the most abundant amino acid in the blood and has many important roles. The amino acid serves as a food source for intestinal cells and is involved in cell division in other parts of the body. Studies show that glutamine can enhance wound healing and help maintain the integrity of the intestinal tract in sick people. Many specialized nutritional formulas contain glutamine in recognition of these functions.

Gluten: A protein in wheat and other grains which is responsible for imparting the elastic quality to breads and other baked goods. Gluten contains another protein fraction, gliadin, that causes damage to the small intestine of people with celiac disease. In this disease, people must avoid wheat, oats, rye, and barley their entire lives.

Goitrogens: Compounds naturally occurring in plant foods which interfere with the production of the thyroid hormones. Goitrogens are present in peanut skins, cabbage, cauliflower, and turnips, but cooking foods destroys them. Theoretically, goitrogens could cause goiter, but the occurrence is unlikely.

Humectants: Substances that enhance moisture retention and prevent drying of foods such as shredded coconut. If shredded coconut didn't contain a humectant, it would lose not only its moisture, but the compounds that produce the characteristic flavor along with it. Humectants form a strong chemical bond with water molecules in the food to retain the moist texture. Other foods to which humectants are commonly added include marshmallows, toaster pastries, and a variety of confections. Common names for humectants include glycerine (glycerol), sorbitol, and propylene glycol.

Inositol: A compound similar to glucose that occurs in nine forms and is found in many plants and animals. In plants, it is present as phytic acid (see *phytic acid*). Although it is not considered to be an essential nutrient, new research suggests that problems in the body's metabolism of this compound may be related to diseases such as diabetes and multiple sclerosis.

Isoflavones: One type of phytoestrogen, found in plant foods, especially in soy products (see *phytoestrogens, genistein*). Both animal and human studies show that increasing the daily intake of soy foods (2 ounces in one human study) alters several parameters related to the menstrual cycle. One of the changes is lengthening the total cycle by an average of one to five days, thereby reducing exposure to endogenous estrogen. Scientists believe that over the course of a lifetime, the exposure to estrogen increases the risk for breast cancer. The high soy intake of some Asian women may account for the lower prevalence of breast cancer in those populations. Good sources of isoflavones include soy flour, with 50 mg of isoflavones in one-half cup; and 1 cup of soy milk, one-half cup tofu, or 1 ounce of soy nuts, all containing 40 mg. Cooked soybeans and textured soy protein are slightly lower at 35 mg in one-half cup.

Lactose: The sugar contained in milk. Many people don't have enough lactase, the enzyme that splits the sugar, and have gastrointestinal problems when they eat foods containing lactose; this condition is called lactose intolerance (LI). Lactase levels are influenced by such factors as genetics, aging, and the condition of the small intestine where the enzyme is made. LI is common in certain ethnic groups including African Americans, Asians, Mexican Americans, Native Americans, and people of Jewish ancestry. People with LI can usually tolerate small amounts of lactose-containing foods spread out through the day. In addition, several special products are available, from milk with predigested lactose to lactase enzyme pills. Milk contains the most lactose, with other dairy products made from milk containing less, and cheese and yogurt generally containing almost no lactose.

Lecithin: A phospholipid that is an important constituent of the cell membrane. The body can synthesize lecithin, and it is naturally occurring in foods. In addition, food manufacturers use lecithin as an emulsifier, which promotes the combining of two compounds that don't mix, such as oil and water. Many people take lecithin supplements for a variety of reasons; it may have a cholesterol-lowering effect at high doses, but high doses can cause gastrointestinal problems.

Lignans: Compounds found in foods, especially flaxseed, soybeans, rye, and berries, which block estrogen activity in cells. Researchers are studying whether lignans' ability to block the hormone can help prevent breast and ovarian cancers. In addition, scientists are investigating a possible role for lignans in preventing heart disease and osteoporosis.

Lignin: An indigestible compound present in the walls of plant cells. For humans, it is a type of insoluble dietary fiber, but because of its toughness, people don't eat much food containing lignin. Lignin occurs in the woody portion of vegetables and seeds of fruits.

Lipoic Acid (thioctic acid): An acid present in meats and spinach which is essential for many animals but not humans, since the body can synthesize the compound. Scientists discovered lipoic acid in 1937 and have learned that it is involved in energy reactions in humans and is closely associated with thiamin. Some researchers believe that it should be considered an important antioxidant, especially in combination with vitamin E. In Germany, lipoic acid has been approved as a painkiller.

Lysine: An essential amino acid naturally present in a variety of foods but generally low in protein from cereal products. Adults who are deficient in lysine experience nausea, vomiting, dizziness, and anemia, while children develop growth failure. Some people have a genetic defect in which the enzyme needed to break down lysine is missing. Symptoms are severe and include gastrointestinal problems, mental retardation, and coma. Lysine was a popular supplement a few years ago, with adherents claiming it was a cure for herpes infection. However, no studies have proven this claim.

Medium-Chain Fatty Acids or **Triglycerides (MCT):** Fatty acids with six to ten carbon atoms, not widely available in foods, that provide fewer calories than long-chain fatty acids. Many nutrition supplements and special products contain MCT instead of regular dietary fat because these fatty acids don't need bile or much enzyme activity for the body to absorb them. This is useful for people who have gastrointestinal disorders that prevent normal fat absorption, including liver disease, Crohn's disease, and celiac disease.

Minerals: Inorganic elements, present in foods in a basic form (see Chapter 1). Below is an alphabetical listing of each essential mineral and a few nonessential ones, which may be considered essential in the future. For each, you'll find basic information on functions and food sources.

Arsenic: A trace mineral which scientists think may be essential for humans, although no RDA has been established. Since ancient times, the fact that arsenic is odorless and tasteless earned it the infamous title as "the king of poisons." However, physicians of the past also used it to treat anorexia, syphilis, asthma, malaria, diabetes, and skin diseases.

Scientists have discovered that minute amounts of arsenic are crucial in maintaining the life span of red blood cells. In animals, arsenic deficiency causes stunted growth, anemia, and death of red blood cells. Seafood and water are the chief dietary sources, but people also get arsenic through inhalation of environmental sources. Toxicity symptoms include weakness, muscle aches, gastrointestinal problems, nerve damage, and changes in skin pigmentation. While large amounts of arsenic are fatal, the amounts normally present in foods are too small to cause toxicity.

Boron: A mineral found in most body tissues and essential to plants. Scientists are studying boron to determine if it's essential for humans. The Food and Nutrition Board of the National Research Council passed over boron when developing the tenth edition of Recommended Dietary Allowances (RDA) in 1989, but current research seems to suggest that boron may be essential. Some investigators believe it plays a major role in mineral metabolism and may be associated with a common chronic disease, osteoporosis. One of the difficulties that researchers encounter in studying this mineral is that it may be required in extremely small amounts, perhaps less than 1 mg per day.

Soon after its discovery, researchers determined that in chicks and rats, several nutrients affected the organisms' response to varying levels of dietary boron. The nutrients they identified included the amino acid methionine, potassium, magnesium, cholecalciferol, manganese, and calcium. These nutrients are involved in one of two functions: maintaining integrity of the cellular membrane and the body's response to hormones. This led researchers to hypothesize that boron may be of nutritional significance when an organism is exposed to stress of nutritional, physiological, or hormonal origin. As such, boron could be involved in the metabolism of macro minerals such as potassium, calcium, and magnesium by affecting the regulatory role of hormones.

One of the leading boron researchers conducted a human study in 1986 to determine the effects of aluminum, magnesium, and boron on mineral metabolism in postmenopausal women, who are most at risk for osteoporosis. Boron supplementation caused a reduction in the levels of calcium and magnesium excreted in urine. Both of these substances are essential for bone mineralization, so increased excretion can compromise bone density. Boron raised the blood levels of two hormones, estradiol-17B and testosterone. Estradiol-17B is a biologically active form of estrogen, and testosterone is its precursor. Currently, estrogen administration is the only treatment documented as being effective in slowing bone calcium loss after menopause.

These same researchers followed with another study which included men. Boron deprivation for nine weeks resulted in decreased blood levels of calcium and vitamin D. Low intake of boron produced increased levels of calcitonin, which is a hormone that regulates calcium concentration in blood, bone, and the amount excreted in the urine. Based on these studies, the Human Nutrition Research Center of the USDA has recommended that boron be established as an essential nutrient. Some scientists have proposed that boron supplementation, in an amount similar to that of a diet high in fruits and vegetables, may help prevent calcium loss and bone demineralization, which lead to osteoporosis.

Boron can be found in many foods of plant origin such as fruits, vegetables, and nuts. Excellent sources include apples, pears, grapes, legumes, and leafy vegetables. Vegetables contain an average of 13 micrograms of boron per gram, while legumes and nuts contain 18 to 23 micrograms per gram. Diets high in animal products tend to be low in boron since meats, fish, and poultry are poor sources, averaging from .16 to .36 micrograms per gram. Dairy products are also poor sources, providing 1.1 micrograms per gram. A surprisingly good source of boron are wines, which provide up to 8.5 micrograms per gram. Based on the studies of boron, one leading researcher has postulated that the requirement may be close 1 to 2 mg per day.

Calcium: The most abundant mineral in the human body, with about 99 percent contained in the bones. The bones support the body structurally and protect soft tissues, and serve as a huge reservoir of calcium, releasing it when needed. While only a small amount of calcium circulates in the blood, its role is vital. Some of its functions involve nerve transmission, muscular contraction including that of the heart, maintenance of cell membranes, and blood clotting.

Because of calcium's vital roles throughout the body, it is released from bone whenever blood levels drop slightly, even at the expense of bone levels. This becomes a problem when calcium intake, or the body's ability to absorb it, doesn't keep pace with the body's needs, such as during growth or as a consequence of the aging process.

A famous researcher once said, "Eat, drink, and be merry, for tomorrow we will all have less bone." His remark may seem flippant, but one fact of aging appears to be a steady decline in bone density for both males and females. The more dense the bone is to start with, however, the less impact this loss will have. In practical terms, males tend to have more bone mass than women, so they don't suffer the ravages of bone loss to the same extent. Osteoporosis, a thinning of the bone and its mineral-based structure, causes bone to become brittle or porous, increasing the likelihood of a fracture.

The new DRI for calcium is set at 1,000 mg for men and women between the ages of 19 and 50 years, and increases to 1,200 mg for adults over age 50. The increase over the 1989 RDAs was the result of experts supporting an increase for post-menopausal women because of the high risk for osteoporosis. Data from population surveys indicate that the mean calcium intake of women ages 19 to 50 is 25 percent below the DRI. Average intakes were even lower in both men and women ages 35 to 50 and people living in poverty.

The best sources of calcium are dairy products: 1 cup of low-fat yogurt or milk contains about 415 mg, half the adult DRI. Dark green leafy vegetables such as broccoli and collard, turnip, and mustard greens contain a substantial amount, with 1 cup of cooked greens averaging 150 mg. However, calcium from vegetable sources is less well absorbed than dairy calcium, because of calcium-binding components found in vegetables. Two health issues may have influenced calcium intake from dairy sources: the high fat content of traditional dairy products and lactose intolerance. The food industry has responded to these concerns by marketing low-fat dairy products, as well as those that are low lactose or lactose free.

Epidemiologists were the first to point to a possible protective effect of calcium against high blood pressure, citing health statistics on regions with a hard water supply. They found lower rates of the disorder, and knowing that calcium levels are higher in hard water paved the way for further clinical trials. Initially, reports of studies using calcium supplements to treat hypertension seemed very promising. Subsequent studies have yielded conflicting results, leading researchers to conclude that calcium's effect on blood pressure may be moderated by the interaction of other minerals. In addition, there may be an individualized response to several of the minerals.

A number of population studies have suggested a protective effect of calcium against colon cancer. A nineteen-year study of almost 2,000 people indicated that calcium intake was significantly lower in those who later developed the disease. Some researchers have suggested that intake must be 1,200 to 2,000 mg to confer calcium's protective effect. However, as with hypertension and calcium, case-controlled studies have been conflicting.

Chloride: An essential ion from the element chlorine, a poisonous gas. The reaction between chlorine gas and sodium produces the negatively charged ion that serves as a major constituent of the fluid outside of cells. In this role, chloride helps to maintain fluid and electrolyte balance. In the stomach, the ion is part of hydrochloric acid, an important player in digestion. A wide variety of foods contain chloride, especially processed foods which contain salt. The estimated minimum requirement for men and women is 750 mg a day, and most Americans have no problem meeting this amount. Some conditions which may deplete chloride include heavy sweating or chronic vomiting and diarrhea.

Chromium: An essential trace mineral which scientists are studying for its prominent role in normal glucose metabolism. Chromium was first found to be required for glucose metabolism in 1959. Later animal studies indicated that chromium works closely with insulin to facilitate uptake and metabolism of glucose in cells, and they defined the mineral as an essential part of an organic complex called the glucose tolerance factor.

Because of difficulty in diagnosing chromium status, the 1989 RDA committee didn't set an RDA for chromium but established the estimated safe and adequate intake at 50 to 200 micrograms. The richest food sources of chromium include whole grains, nuts, organ meats, and brewer's yeast. Good sources include fruits, vegetables, bran, and some breakfast cereals, but most foods provide only 10 to 15 percent of the minimum level. Interestingly, beer and wine are both good sources of chromium.

From intake surveys, nutritionists estimate that more than 90 percent of the U.S. population isn't consuming an adequate amount. In terms of toxicity, the NRC reports that the form of chromium present in foods poses virtually no potential for negative effects. Several factors can cause a suboptimal intake: stress, trauma, and strenuous exercise can all deplete body stores. Additionally, researchers reported that a high-sugar diet can deplete body stores of chromium.

Researchers have also found that chromium enhances the metabolism of sugar in about 85 percent of people who are slightly glucose intolerant. They theorize that this effect indicates that these individuals are chromium deficient. Glucose intolerance is thought to be an early stage or sign of Type 2 diabetes. This type of diabetes develops in adults and is caused by the secretion of ineffective insulin, in contrast to Type 1 diabetes, in which the pancreas can't make insulin.

Copper: A mineral found to be essential for many animals and even some lower species. Although scientists have long known that humans require copper, new research is pointing to a preventive role in cardiovascular disease and cancer. A 1928 study of rats was the first to suggest that copper is essential for the formation of hemoglobin. Less than forty years later, researchers reported defects of the bone and central nervous system in pigs fed a copper-deficient diet. They noted that these defects were similar to those seen in domestic animals grazing on copper-deficient soil: swayback in lambs and osteoporosis in cattle.

Copper is present in all tissues but concentrated in the liver, brain, heart, and kidney. Its major role in the body is in copper-containing enzymes which are involved in important chemical reactions. About 90 percent of copper in the blood is present as a copper complex, ceruloplasmin. This molecule is required to change the oxidation state of iron, the chemical reaction needed for the body to use iron to make hemoglobin. In the same way, copper affects iron absorption and the process of freeing iron from liver stores, making it available to the body.

Another important copper enzyme helps in the formation of connective tissue. Because of this function, copper deficiency produces damaging changes in heart tissue and bone disorders in animals and humans. One form of the enzyme, superoxide dismutase, contains copper. This enzyme is present in most tissues and defends against free radical damage. Yet another copper enzyme helps make melanin, and this affects normal pigmentation when deficient.

Two genetic diseases are related to copper. In Menkes syndrome, intestinal cells absorb copper but are unable to release it into the blood when it's needed. Symptoms include unusual hair texture, which is related to copper's function in the formation of keratin, and stunted development. Because absorption is normal, oral copper supplements are not effective. Instead, copper must be injected, but brain levels of copper can't be restored, and tissue damage continues there. In contrast, Wilson disease represents a copper toxicity. The absence of an enzyme needed to form ceruloplasmin, which binds copper to allow for removal, causes the liver and brain to store toxic levels. The first symptoms are those of liver disease.

In the United States, hospital physicians have reported copper deficiency in premature infants on intravenous feeding. Because of insufficient data, copper doesn't have an RDA. However, the RDA committee set an Estimated Safe and Adequate Daily Dietary Intake (ESADDI) of 1.5 to 3 mg for adults. To put this in perspective, human breast milk contains 0.3 mg per liter. The Food and Drug Administration estimated that, from 1982 to 1986, Americans' daily copper intake averaged 0.9 mg and 1.2 mg for women and men, respectively.

While it seems that Americans may not be getting enough copper, many scientists believe that the body efficiently absorbs more copper when intake is low, reducing the incidence of deficiency. Nutrient interaction may increase the risk of low copper absorption. Researchers have reported that in animals high intakes of zinc, ascorbic acid, and iron seriously affect copper status. Since these are common supplements, the same interaction can occur in humans. Recent studies have shown that these nutrients, particularly zinc, can impair copper status in humans. Fructose and sucrose can potentially interact with copper.

Copper is widely distributed in most foods. The most concentrated sources include organ meats and seafood. Liver contains 6 mg of copper in a 3-ounce serving, and shrimp has approximately half that level. Excellent plant sources include legumes, nuts, dried fruits, and whole grains. The dairy group is notable by its absence from this list. Milk checks in at a scant .002 mg per half-cup. The best contributors are plant products, which provide about 62 percent of the copper in the average U.S. diet. Copper is highly toxic, with as little as 10 to 30 mg of copper causing physical distress, and doses above 500 mg fatal. As proof of copper's toxicity, poisoning with this mineral was a traditional method of suicide in India.

Since copper is needed for the formation of heart and blood vessel tissues as well as enzymes which protect against oxidation, researchers are investigating a possible role in chronic diseases such as heart disease and cancer. Numerous animal studies have indicated that copper deficiency can produce heart disease. Most recently, clinicians have identified fifty physiological similarities between people with heart disease and copper-deficient animals. The similarities include glucose intolerance, high blood cholesterol, abnormal electrocardiograms, and hypertension.

Scientists have also proposed that copper's role in the superoxide dismutase enzyme, which grabs free radicals, may confer a possible protective benefit against cancer. Some evidence for this comes from animal studies showing that rats fed supplemental copper had lower rates of tumors when exposed to cancer-causing agents.

Fluoride: An essential trace mineral contained in higher amounts in bones, teeth, thyroid gland, and skin. The latest DRI committee bumped fluoride up to essential status with its latest revision. Studies have shown for many years that the mineral helps protect children's teeth against dental caries.

Fluoride forms fluoroapatite in bones and teeth which hardens tooth enamel and makes bone structure more stable. Most Americans get fluoride in their water supply, and others get it in beverages made from fluoridated water and foods grown in soil containing the mineral. Fluoride is potentially toxic, with its safety range being the most narrow of all the minerals. High levels can cause the teeth to mottle, and single doses over 5 grams have caused death.

Iodine: A mineral determined to be essential in 1918 when two scientists discovered that goiter could be cured in some cases by small amounts of supplemental iodine. Their cure was so dramatic that this discovery led to a public health measure which persists to this day of fortifying table salt with iodine.

Simple goiter refers to enlargement of the thyroid gland due to deficiency of the mineral, whereas toxic goiter occurs in cases of glandular hyperfunction. Certain foods, which contain antithyroxin compounds called goitrogens (see *goitrogens*) have been used in large quantities to produce goiter in experimental animals. These foods include cabbage, turnips, and rutabagas; however, it is unlikely that humans would eat sufficient quantities to precipitate goiter. Goiters are rare in this country these days, but students of the health professions are familiar with textbook photographs of grapefruit-sized glands horribly altering the necks and faces of afflicted patients.

It appears that iodine's only physiological function is to serve as a constituent of thyroxine and other compounds released by the thyroid gland, which regulates cellular energy transduction and other important functions. Thyroid activity is controlled by thyroid stimulating hormone (TSP), which is secreted by the pituitary. When blood levels of thyroxine are low, TSP steps up the thyroid's release of the hormone, resulting in an increase in the size of the gland's cells. When iodine is deficient, producing chronically low blood levels of thyroxine, thyroid enlargement occurs because TSP continues to stimulate thyroid cells.

The functions of the thyroid hormones are extremely important, ranging from the regulation of oxygen consumption and metabolic rate to profound effects on growth, via its role in protein synthesis. Additionally, early studies administering thyroxine into test animals demonstrated an increased activity of several key growth enzymes.

The Recommended Dietary Allowance (RDA) for iodine is 150 micrograms for both adult men and women. The amount of environmental iodine varies by region in the United States. Coastal areas are higher in available iodine because of higher consumption of seafood and exposure to oceanic water, both directly and through the mist blowing from the water. As one moves further inland, iodine content in plant and animal foods decreases but still varies depending on several influences. Chief among these are the geological attributes of an area, along with fertilization and farming practices.

Another very significant source, because of their high salt content addition, are commercially prepared foods. Another contributor to high levels in commercial products is the use of iodine compounds in processing, such as dough oxidizers in baked goods. In addition, dairy products tend to pick up the mineral via disinfectants used in various aspects of the dairy industry as well as additives in animal feed.

Iron: An essential nutrient that most people associate with anemia. In the United States and Canada, experts estimate that 20 percent of all women and 3 percent of men have depleted iron stores and another 8 percent and 1 percent, respectively, have anemia. The human body contains about 5.5 ounces of iron for every pound of fat-free body weight. Most of the body's iron is connected to protein compounds, with hemoglobin being the predominant form and myoglobin a distant second. Both of these proteins carry or hold oxygen: hemoglobin carries this vital element to the body's tissues, and myoglobin serves as the oxygen reservoir in muscle cells. All cells require oxygen in order to combine with the carbon and hydrogen atoms released in the breakdown of energy nutrients. In addition to this critical function, iron is also involved in several enzyme systems which are important in energy metabolism.

The amount of iron in the body is tightly regulated by iron absorption in the intestine; absorption, in turn, is influenced by body stores of iron. The amount and chemical form of iron in food and the presence of dietary factors either enhance or inhibit absorption. One dietary factor which enhances iron absorption is ascorbic acid. Just the simple addition of orange juice to a meal will increase iron absorption. When iron stores are low, absorption is increased, as during times of increased need such as pregnancy.

There are two chemical forms of iron, heme and nonheme iron. Heme iron, found exclusively in animal products, is much more absorbable than nonheme iron, which is contained in vegetable sources. When a nonheme iron source is combined with a heme source, absorption of the nonheme is enhanced. Even under the best circumstances, iron absorption from foods tends to be around 10 percent.

Well-known inhibitors of iron absorption include phytates, bran, polyphenols in tea, and various medications such as antacids. Phytates, found in vegetables and grains, are insoluble compounds which bind essential minerals such as calcium, phosphorus, iron, and zinc, rendering them unabsorbable. Other inhibitors probably chelate minerals the same way to decrease absorption of iron. Inhibition of absorption affects mostly nonheme iron, reflecting tight control of nonheme iron absorption. The absorption of iron from a meal decreases as the amount of iron present increases.

People at risk for iron-deficiency anemia include urban dwellers and the rural poor. On a positive note, the rate of anemia has dropped in low-income children in the United States. The causes of iron-deficiency anemia can be varied and include inadequate dietary intake, blood loss, and parasitic infection. Blood loss normally occurs in menstruating women and is the primary cause of iron deficiency in 20 percent of North American women.

The RDA for iron is 15 mg for adult women and 10 mg for men. Iron is fairly widely distributed in foods available to most Americans. Good sources, especially of heme iron, are meat products, particularly red meats. Eggs, vegetables, and grains contain fair amounts of nonheme iron which isn't as well absorbed. Iron-fortified breakfast cereals are among the highest available dietary sources of iron. In terms of toxicity, iron hasn't been shown to cause detrimental effects at levels of 25 to 75 mg per day from food sources. However, close to 2,000 cases of iron poisoning are reported annually in the United States, primarily young children accidentally taking adult iron supplements.

Magnesium: An essential mineral that scientists have recently linked to high blood pressure and heart disease. The first evidence for its essentiality came in 1936 when scientists discovered that rats deprived of magnesium developed tetany. It wasn't until 1964, however, that magnesium deficiency was demonstrated in humans by using volunteers. The subjects developed personality changes, muscle tremor, lack of coordination, and gastrointestinal problems after three months. The deficiency also caused changes in calcium and potassium balance, with blood levels of these minerals dropping along with magnesium levels.

Most of the magnesium in the body, about 60 percent, resides in bone, with the other 40 percent contained in muscle and other soft tissue. It functions in many cellular processes as part of a complex with the body's form of energy currency, adenosine triphosphate (ATP), and as an activator of over 300 enzymes. Some of the reactions in which magnesium plays a role include energy metabolism and the transmission of the genetic code. In addition, scientists believe that magnesium outside the cell is involved in the transmission of nerve impulses.

The DRI for men and women under fifty years of age is 420 mg and 320 mg, respectively. Magnesium is widely available in the food supply, occurring in most unprocessed foods. The best sources include nuts, legumes, and whole grains. Unfortunately, more than 80 percent can be lost in the milling process of cereal grains when the outer layers of the grain and the germ within are removed. Dark green vegetables are good sources, with a one-half-cup serving of broccoli providing 47 mg. However, meat and dairy products are low in this essential mineral, and, in combination with the losses from processing, low or marginal intakes may occur.

People taking magnesium supplements don't appear to suffer any toxic effects if their kidneys are functioning properly. When kidneys have lost their ability to excrete, high levels of magnesium can be retained and produce toxic effects with symptoms of nausea, vomiting, and dangerously low blood pressure. These can progress to adverse changes in heartbeat and the central nervous system, leading to respiratory failure and cardiac arrest. Toxicity is also possible in people who are using magnesium-containing drugs. However, over-the-counter preparations such as antacids and laxatives which contain magnesium are thought to be safe.

Lower rates of high blood pressure and heart disease among rural dwellers was the first clue that magnesium might protect against these scourges of civilization. Hard water supplies are generally high in mineral content such as calcium and magnesium; in contrast, soft water supplies in cities are nearly devoid of these minerals. More direct evidence comes from a few studies that reported that magnesium deficiency makes the walls of blood vessels constrict more readily, thereby raising blood pressure. Magnesium also appears to function in the maintenance of normal heart rhythm during attacks of ischemia, a transitory lack of oxygen to heart tissue. Scientists believe that this role may explain the lower rate of sudden cardiac death rates in rural areas where the population has a hard water supply high in magnesium.

Manganese: A trace mineral researchers discovered in the 1930s determined to be essential to almost all animals. Most consumers confuse this nutrient with another mineral that starts with an "m," magnesium. The two minerals are similar in their chemistry, although manganese is required in very small amounts, making it a trace mineral, though every bit as essential to human life.

Initially, scientists had difficulty determining the mineral's role in humans. Although manganese was known to activate several enzyme systems, other similar minerals, especially magnesium, were equally as effective. Researchers have found two enzymes dependent solely on manganese, one of which is superoxide dismutase, involved as a scavenger of free radicals. The enzymes are located in the mitochondria of cells, often called the cells' power plants because of energy production occurring in these structures. Consequently, tissues which are high in mitochondria, such as liver, kidney, and pancreas, have high concentrations of manganese.

For many years, nutritionists believed that humans absorbed only 5 percent of dietary manganese. Now it is thought that absorption is dependent on dietary intake, but the actual amount remains unknown. Part of the problem with studying this elusive mineral lies with the lack of a practical method to assess a person's manganese status. Animal studies show that blood manganese levels reflect the body's manganese status, but in mineral-depleted human subjects no changes appear in blood levels. One aspect of manganese absorption which is known is its similarity to that of iron. It has been speculated that since this similarity causes competition for absorption, problems can arise: when one mineral is present in high amounts, absorption of the other will be inhibited.

Manganese deficiency in animals produces congenital mal-
formations, growth retardation, poor reproduction, abnormal
development of cartilage and bone, and defects in glucose tolerance. Human deficiency of manganese is virtually unknown
because of its abundant supply in most plant products. However,
one reported case was of a man with a vitamin K deficiency
who was fed a purified diet which did not contain manganese.
Since then, formulas used to feed patients parenterally (via
veins) have the mineral added. Manganese toxicity was somewhat common among miners working with manganic oxide
through inhalation of the dust. Symptoms of toxicity are similar to viral encephalitis accompanied by body tremors.

Manganese doesn't have an RDA; instead it has an
Estimated Safe and Adequate Daily Dietary Intake (ESADDI)
set at a range of 2 to 5 mg. The new DRIs will update manganese
recommendations in the coming year. Good sources of the mineral include whole grains and cereal products. Vegetables and
fruits are fair sources, and dairy, meat, and poultry are considered poor sources of manganese. Tea is an unusually rich source
of the mineral.

Some intriguing studies have been done in the past five
years. One study, in which fourteen women were fed a low-
manganese diet, reported an increase in blood glucose during a
glucose tolerance test. In addition, the low-manganese diet
caused higher menstrual losses of manganese, calcium, and
iron, as well as lower total hemoglobin. Another study showed
that blood manganese levels were lower in patients with certain
types of epilepsy, a finding which may correlate to rat studies in
which manganese deficiency increases the risk for convulsions.
Manganese's role in human immunity is another area awaiting
further exploration, as some studies suggest that it stimulates
certain components of the immune response. In addition, animals fed a manganese-deficient diet had decreased levels of
important immunoglobulins.

Molybdenum: A trace mineral that functions in enzyme systems. Molybdenum is a relative latecomer to the nutrition scene. However, numerous animal studies and a few human studies have quite dramatically shown the essentiality of this mineral.

The first clue that molybdenum was an important nutrient, possibly essential to human life, came in 1953 with the discovery of the enzyme xanthine oxidase, which contains the mineral. At first, it appeared that molybdenum was only essential for chickens. The first indication of molybdenum's significance in humans involved a patient on long-term total parenteral nutrition (TPN). Patients on TPN receive a solution containing all essential nutrients intravenously as their only source of nutrition. In that first case, the patient developed a number of symptoms which included intolerance to amino acids, irritability, and finally coma. When molybdenum was added to the solution, the patient began to improve.

The only other situation in which molybdenum deficiency has developed is in a rare genetic metabolic defect in which two enzymes dependent on the mineral are deficient. Patients with this defect suffer from a severe neurologic disorder and mental retardation. The functions of molybdenum primarily involve its role as an enzyme cofactor in three enzymes which catalyze the addition of a hydrogen and oxygen group (hydroxylation) of many compounds. The mineral may also be involved in reactions involving steroid metabolism.

The 1989 RDA still covers molybdenum with an ESADDI of 75 to 250 micrograms. The most important food sources of molybdenum include milk, beans, breads, and cereals. However, the mineral content of food varies widely depending on environmental growing conditions, which may negate the usefulness of values listed in food composition tables. Dietary surveys indicate that daily intakes in the United States average 180 micrograms. Of more concern is possible toxicity because of the antagonism between molybdenum and copper. Researchers have reported adverse effects of high environmental levels of the mineral in a province of the former Soviet Union. In addition to excessive urinary losses of copper, the symptoms included a syndrome resembling gout.

Nickel: A trace mineral essential to some animals, but scientists have not yet declared it essential for humans. Researchers believe that the mineral may be involved as a cofactor in many enzyme systems, just as other essential minerals. In animals, nickel deficiency causes stunted growth, decline in blood synthesis, and changes in levels of several trace minerals in the liver. Of interest is nickel's effect on iron absorption, but nickel also appears to affect the metabolism of several minerals.

Most nickel in the human body is concentrated in skin and bone marrow. Dietary intake for most people averages .3 to .6 mg per day. The best sources include nuts, dried beans and peas, chocolate, and grains. Nickel is toxic at high levels, causing degeneration of heart, brain, lung, and liver tissue.

Phosphorus: An essential mineral needed in amounts equivalent to that for calcium; the body prefers a one-to-one ratio of these two vital minerals. While phosphorus is needed in relatively large amounts, there has been a growing concern that Americans may consume too much phosphorus.

Phosphorus is the second most plentiful mineral in the body, with 85 percent of it combined in a crystalline matrix of calcium in bones and teeth. However, in the blood, the concentration of phosphorus is half that of calcium. Salt forms of the mineral act as buffers to maintain the proper acid-to-base balance of cellular fluids. A critical function is as a component of each cell's genetic material, making phosphorus essential for growth and repair of tissues. Another key function is as the main energy currency of the body in adenosine triphosphate (ATP). In a less active role, phosphorus contributes to cellular membranes as a part of the phospholipid compounds which make up these structures.

The updated DRI for phosphorus is 700 mg for men and women, and Americans obtain most of their intake from animal products and processed foods. Phosphate additives are important in the food industry, appearing in a myriad of products in which they perform various functions. As people increasingly rely on processed foods, excessive phosphorus intake has become a concern.

The reason for concern relates to several effects which occur when the phosphorus-to-calcium ratio exceeds the ideal of one to one. Early studies showed that low calcium-to-phosphorus ratios (one to four) resulted in enlarged parathyroid glands, low serum calcium levels, and loss of bone mineral mass. In a more recent study, women who were fed a one-to-four diet for four weeks had increased levels of the parathyroid hormone (PTH). Persistently elevated PTH levels cause a net loss of calcium and phosphorus from bone, making it more susceptible to fractures from osteoporosis, a bone-thinning disease of the elderly.

Other human studies have shown that meals containing a high phosphate level and low amounts of calcium increase calcium excretion. Researchers have theorized that the phosphates form insoluble complexes with calcium, rendering it unabsorbable. In addition, phosphorus absorption tends to depress calcium absorption due to the action of the hormone calcitonin. Over a period of years, it is thought that this imbalance of phosphorus to calcium and resulting reduction in calcium absorption can also increase the risk for osteoporosis.

Most Americans don't meet the RDA for calcium, and this fact together with the increasing presence of phosphate additives gives rise for concern. Recent national surveys confirm that Americans consume far more phosphorus than calcium, with one reporting the calcium-to-phosphorus intake at one to one and a half.

The most significant source of phosphate additives are carbonated beverages, consumption of which has witnessed a huge increase in the past ten years. Studies from the 1980s estimated that Americans consume 400 mg of phosphate additives daily, and more recently researchers have proposed that this quantity may be greatly underestimated and is closer to 800 mg.

Potassium: An essential mineral familiar to many older people because of the use of diuretics, drugs which deplete the body's supply of potassium. Potassium is essential to the life of the body's cells: it is one of two minerals present in the highest amount within each cell. One of its most basic functions is to maintain the proper balance of water and other minerals, the electrolytes. It is by this function that potassium maintains the integrity of the cell itself. Another more dramatic function is in sustaining the heartbeat. Sudden deaths associated with fasting, diarrhea, and starvation are probably caused by heart failure induced by potassium deficiency.

Potassium deficiency among older individuals arises from the use of diuretic drugs. Diuretics are used to reduce the volume of fluid in the body, which is helpful in people with high blood pressure and some types of heart failure. Certain types of diuretics deplete potassium as they increase fluid excretion. People taking these drugs usually need to increase their intake of high-potassium foods or take potassium supplements. Others at risk for deficiency are those who sweat profusely on a consistent basis, such as during strenuous physical activity.

Another group of people for whom potassium is a concern are those with kidney disease. However, the problem here is not too little potassium but rather too much. The kidney normally filters the blood and excretes excess amounts of either water or minerals. At a certain stage of kidney failure, the ability to remove excess potassium is diminished or lost altogether. Just as potassium is crucial for maintaining a normal heartbeat, an excess can cause erratic beating and lead to cardiac arrest. People at this stage of kidney disease must carefully control their dietary intake of foods containing potassium.

An RDA has not been established for potassium, but the 1989 RDA committee set the estimated minimum requirement at 2 grams for adults. Among food sources of potassium, fruits and vegetables rank the highest, followed by fresh meats. However, within these broad food groups, there is a wide variation in potassium content. Excellent sources include orange juice, bananas, and potatoes, with values for standard servings of 496, 451, and 844 mg, respectively.

Epidemiologic studies from the mid-1970s suggested that the mineral exerted a protective effect against high blood pressure. Populations consuming higher amounts of foods containing potassium tended to have a lower prevalence of the disorder. This led researchers to conduct more controlled animal studies, which subsequently yielded conflicting results. One early theory proposed that rather than potassium exerting an independent effect, the ratio of potassium to sodium in the diet influenced blood pressure. The current thinking is that potassium's effect on blood pressure is probably part of a complex interplay among various essential minerals, such as sodium, chloride, and magnesium.

Selenium: An essential trace mineral, which scientists didn't identify as essential until 1957. A clue to its discovery was its characteristic garliclike odor, although the first breakthrough came more recently when scientists elucidated the nature of the selenoenzyme. Since then, selenium has kept researchers busy with a myriad of claims and queries. The 1989 RDAs included selenium because of its relationship to the prevention of chronic disease.

The function of selenium is interrelated with that of vitamin E: The status of one of these nutrients affects the requirement for the other. Selenium's main function is as an active part of the glutathione peroxidase enzyme, which consists of four subunits, each containing selenium. This enzyme catalyzes the breakdown of a specific oxygen radical, thereby protecting cell membranes from oxidative damage. A growing area of interest is selenium's interaction with many other nutrients, including the specific amino acids, protein, fats, vitamins, other minerals, and some heavy metals.

Geographic differences in selenium content of plants and soil have stimulated scientific research on the possible action of this mineral in cancer prevention. New Zealand is an important area with active ongoing research because of its many soil types containing varying amounts of selenium. In the United States, research over the past twenty years has clearly demonstrated an inverse correlation between cancer and selenium levels in soil and crops. In 1976, a study of several U.S. cities showed that higher blood levels of selenium were associated with lower cancer mortality.

Silicon: A trace mineral essential for chickens and rats, in which deficiency causes growth retardation and abnormal skeletal development. Some scientists believe that this mineral may be essential for humans as well, but it is not currently covered by the RDA. Interesting studies have suggested that silicon may play a role in atherosclerosis, with reports that when levels in a blood vessel wall are low, atherosclerosis progresses. In addition, other studies have shown that silicon in drinking water may lower blood cholesterol. Many foods contain the mineral, and good sources include unrefined grains and cereals and root vegetables. Other sources include over-the-counter antacids containing magnesium silicate, and processed foods containing silicates as food additives to prevent caking and foaming.

Sodium: A major mineral essential to life, and valued throughout history, even used as currency. More recently, this essential mineral has come under scrutiny for its possible role in high blood pressure, a major risk factor for both heart attack and stroke.

As a part of table salt, sodium chloride, sodium accounts for 40 percent of the compound. In the body, sodium is the major mineral of fluid outside of cells, and, as such, it determines the amount of fluid in that compartment. Sodium also plays a key role in the regulation of acid-base balance and concentration of the blood. Other functions involve influencing muscle contraction and transport of compounds across the cell membrane.

In addition to dietary sodium intake, the environment affects sodium levels because sodium is lost in sweat. In high temperatures and humid conditions, a person engaged in heavy physical exertion can lose significant amounts of sodium. Other causes for significant losses include chronic diarrhea and kidney disease.

An RDA is not established for sodium, but the estimated minimum requirement is 115 mg of sodium or 300 mg of salt. Processed foods are high in salt and sodium, which are used as additives, but considering that even whole foods such as milk contains 123 mg, it is clear that Americans consume substantially more sodium than needed. A landmark study found that only 10 percent of the salt in American diets arises from the natural salt content of foods, with another 15 percent added in preparation or at the table, and 75 percent from salt and other sodium additives used in manufacturer processing. Because of this fact, diets which emphasize processed foods are the highest in sodium content, and diets high in fruits and vegetables are lower in salt.

Excessive intake of sodium chloride increases the amount of water retained in the body in addition to pulling water from cells. The result is edema and high blood pressure, which may occur in some individuals. It is the possible relationship to the development of high blood pressure, also termed hypertension, that accounts for the dietary restriction of salt recommended by most health agencies. Hypertension is a major risk factor for heart attack and stroke, and a government survey reported that 24 percent of Americans have this condition. The 1989 RDA committee recommended that sodium intake should be limited to 2,400 mg or less daily.

The difficulty has been that not all people respond to high salt intakes with an increase in blood pressure. Some studies have shown that a reduction in salt intake can increase blood pressure in some people. In epidemiologic studies, the results have been just as conflicting, with some showing that as salt intake increases, blood pressure increases, and still others showing no correlation.

One explanation for the controversy is the well-accepted theory that some people are sensitive to sodium's effect on blood pressure, while others are not. Because there is no reliable test to determine salt sensitivity, a study would normally include participants of both persuasions with conflicting results.

Adding to the confusion and growing concern is a large prospective study published last year of 2,581 mild hypertensive men. They found that men with the lowest urinary excretion of sodium had a significantly higher risk of heart attack and total cardiovascular disease compared to men with the highest sodium excretion. Urinary sodium excretion ostensibly reflects sodium intake. Another study found that while sodium restriction enhances the efficacy of some antihypertensive agents, when used with a certain type called calcium channel blockers, blood pressure increased. Even with the conflicting studies and concerns, most health agencies recommend that Americans cut down on salt intake.

Sulfur: A mineral that is present in all cells but is concentrated in cartilage, skin, and hair. The mineral isn't essential on its own, but it is part of thiamin and two essential amino acids, methionine and cysteine. Along with other minerals present in body fluids, it helps to maintain the proper balance. If a person eats foods that contain methionine and cysteine, they will have adequate sulfur.

Zinc: An essential trace mineral needed by humans, animals, and plants. Although scientists had reported zinc deficiency in lab animals, it wasn't until the early 1960s that they recognized its importance to humans. The seminal research took place in areas of the Middle East where an American physician studied young males whose growth and sexual maturation had seemingly ceased. The physician was astounded to find out that boys who appeared to be about eight years old were actually sixteen or seventeen.

The diet in the affected areas consisted mainly of cereals with little or no animal protein. While the researchers theorized that the symptoms could be due to zinc deficiency, analysis of the diet yielded a marginal, but probably adequate, level of zinc. However, they still suspected zinc deficiency, and after they gave the boys zinc supplements, the symptoms, which included severe growth retardation and lack of sexual development, dramatically improved. This led to the discovery that, while the dietary level of zinc was adequate, the mineral is poorly absorbed from plant products. The chief villain in the Middle Eastern diet was the presence of phytic acid in the grain used to make bread.

In the intestinal tract, phytic acid forms insoluble complexes with essential minerals such as calcium, phosphorus, iron, and zinc, rendering them unabsorbable and eventually excreted. The phytate structure can be split by an enzyme called phytase which nullifies its binding capability, rendering the minerals available to the body. This enzyme is present in yeast, liver, malt, and seeds. Unfortunately for the zinc-deficient young males, their staple food was unleavened bread, which is prepared without yeast.

In the body, zinc performs a countless number of critical functions, primarily through its role in the formation or action of more than seventy enzymes. Some of these enzymes control vital functions including the maintenance of acid-base balance, excretion of toxic ammonia, production of hydrochloric acid needed for digestion, protein digestion, detoxification of alcohol, and formation of collagen in wound healing. In addition, zinc is critical in reproduction, growth and sexual development, and appetite by affecting the senses of taste and smell.

The RDA for zinc is 15 mg per day for men and 12 mg for women. The body tightly regulates zinc balance because of its important functions: when zinc stores are low, more zinc will be absorbed. Similarly, when zinc stores are high, more zinc will be excreted. The best dietary sources of zinc are high-protein foods in which the protein is readily available to the body. The average American obtains roughly 70 percent of his zinc from animal products. Cereals are the major source of zinc from plant products, but high phytate levels make zinc less available. Meat, liver, eggs, and seafood are high in zinc, with a 3.5-ounce serving of ground beef averaging 7 mg.

Other essential minerals, especially iron, tend to compete with zinc for absorption. Many studies have documented the zinc-iron competition, which may be significant when a person takes a high-dose supplement of either mineral. Apart from interfering with iron absorption, zinc supplementation may produce its own problems. Zinc toxicity has been known to occur, although it is uncommon. It has been documented in hospitalized patients receiving either long-term zinc therapy or intravenous nutrition. In addition, clinicians have reported toxic effects at levels of 2,000 mg or less per day.

Some of the more exciting research discoveries involve zinc's role in gene expression. Zinc appears to be required for the proper folding of protein strands in DNA replication. Researchers have proposed that the protein strands, which are the first step in replication, fold around a zinc atom, forming a separate structure, termed "zinc fingers." Another important research direction has been zinc's role in immune functions. Studies have shown that several key cells involved in immune response depend on zinc.

Monosodium Glutamate (MSG): A flavor enhancer widely used in the food industry. MSG is the monosodium salt of the amino acid, glutamic acid. In the human mouth, it has a unique ability to enhance the perception of other flavors. Recent research indicates that MSG stimulates a unique flavor separate from the accepted tastes of sweet, salty, bitter, and sour, called umami (see *umami*).

Most studies of MSG has been directed at the purported adverse reaction which occurs in a minority of individuals called "Chinese Restaurant Syndrome." The syndrome derives its name from the fact that Asian cuisine often uses the compound liberally. The symptoms include burning sensation, throbbing headache, facial flushing, and chest pain. Over the years, many studies have been done with conflicting results. The current thinking is that a small number of people may have a sensitivity to MSG and do indeed experience an adverse reaction. Although it is widely used in the food industry, it is not used in infant foods because studies have shown that high doses cause brain cell destruction in developing mice.

While the final verdict is not yet in on a possible role of MSG in Chinese Restaurant Syndrome, experts advise people who believe they are affected to avoid the compound. Additionally, because studies have shown that carbohydrate-containing meals may prevent the reaction, sensitive individuals should eat plenty of rice when enjoying Asian cuisine.

Nutriceuticals: Substances that supposedly offer health benefits, but currently are not recognized by the FDA.

Olestra™: Trade name for sucrose polyester (SP), an unabsorbable compound which mimics many qualities of dietary fat. The FDA recently permitted the use of this artificial fat in snack foods. Foods that contain SP must include a warning label that points to possible side effects that may include diarrhea, cramps, and other intestinal problems. In addition, SP-containing products must also be fortified with fat soluble nutrients, since these may be excreted along with the compound.

Studies of SP's effects on nutrient absorption have been of keen interest to experts and consumers alike with the introduction of this new food additive. The nutrients to be added to SP-containing foods include the fat soluble vitamins, A, D, E, and K. Consumers watching their weight benefit from the nutrient profile of foods containing SP: chips contain zero fat and only 60 calories while the traditional product provides 150 calories and 10 grams of fat. An added bonus is a blood cholesterol–lowering effect demonstrated in several studies. Other fat substitutes on the market have not fared well; one reason is their inability to withstand the heat of frying. Additionally, those substitutes don't mimic fat's characteristics as well as SP, and they are not calorie free, as is SP.

Oxalate: A naturally occurring salt present in a variety of plant foods. Oxalates interfere with calcium absorption and are the basis for a common type of kidney stone. People who have had oxalate kidney stones often follow a low-oxalate diet, and drinking plenty of fluids, usually 3 to 4 liters daily, may be even more important. Rich sources of oxalate include rhubarb, beets, berries, spinach, endive, green beans, sweet potato, swiss chard, collard greens, nuts, tea, and cocoa. In addition, a recent study showed that different types of beverages influenced the development of kidney stones in women. Beverages showing a protective effect included regular and decaffeinated coffee, tea, and wine, while grapefruit juice significantly increased risk for kidney stones.

Pangamic Acid: A compound present in apricot pits, rice, liver, and yeast. When scientists first discovered pangamic acid, they believed it to be a B vitamin and called it vitamin B_{15}. The reasons for their mistake included the compound's wide variety of physiologic effects, including enhanced oxygen uptake and adaptation to oxygen deprivation and strenuous activity. However, subsequent studies have not shown a deficiency disease when the compound is missing in the diet.

Phytic Acid (phytate): A nonnutrient compound found in plant seeds, grain husks, and legumes, consisting of a ring of phosphorus groups. It has the ability to bind other compounds and prevent their absorption. This can have negative health consequences when phytate grabs essential minerals. Studies show that phytate binds calcium, zinc, iron, copper, and magnesium, and forms an insoluble complex with them which the intestine can't absorb and so excretes into the feces.

On a more positive health note, phytate may act as an antioxidant to protect against the oxidative damage which can cause cancer; it may also prevent activation of cancer-causing genes. To date, this evidence has come only from in vitro studies.

Phytochemicals: Nonnutrient compounds in plant foods that are biologically active in the body; includes a variety of compounds including phytoestrogens and plant pigments like lycopene.

Phytoestrogens (phytosterols): Compounds exerting weak hormonelike effects, found in various plant foods, especially soy foods. Soy foods contain one type of phytoestrogen, isoflavones, and most of the studies have been done with these compounds (see *isoflavones, genistein*).

Protease Inhibitors: A group of substances present in a variety of plant foods which can inhibit protein-splitting enzymes. The most famous protease inhibitor is trypsin inhibitor, found in soybeans and other legumes. The compound could prevent utilization of the protein by a person eating the bean, but heat destroys the inhibitor. Recent research suggests that protease inhibitors may also suppress enzyme activity in cancer cells and slow their growth.

Psyllium: A seed from certain plant species which contains large amounts of soluble fiber. Studies have shown that soluble fiber is effective in lowering blood cholesterol and regulating blood glucose level. In addition, soluble fiber exerts positive effects in the gastrointestinal tract, including the generation of short-chain fatty acids (see *short chain fatty acids*), which may help prevent colon cancer, and adding bulk to feces. Large amounts of psyllium can cause gastrointestinal problems such as anorexia, gas, and pain. In addition, psyllium can interfere with the absorption of essential minerals.

Purines: A large group of nitrogen-containing compounds naturally occurring in foods and produced by the body as a result of protein digestion. High levels of purine in the body may influence the development of kidney stones and gout. Doctors prescribe low-purine diets to lower uric acid levels in the blood which may prevent recurrence of kidney stones or treat gout, although it's not clear if the diet is effective. Foods to avoid include red meats, organ meats, anchovies, sardines, and meat extracts.

Quercetin: A yellow pigment found in onion skin, tea, red rose, asparagus, grapefruit, and lemon juice that has antioxidant abilities. It is probably the compound responsible for grapefruit's ability to enhance the absorption of drugs in the stomach, and studies have shown a protection against ulcers. Recent lab studies show that feeding rats grapefruit juice reduces the rate of experimentally induced cancers.

Radiolytic Products: Chemicals formed in foods exposed to ionizing radiation. The FDA has approved the use of irradiation for certain foods and considers the process a food additive. Irradiated foods must indicate so on the label, and the only exception is commercially prepared foods that contain irradiated ingredients such as spices. The benefits of food irradiation include the destruction of harmful microorganisms, insects, and the parasitic worm which may infest pork. In addition, irradiation prevents spoilage by inhibiting the growth of sprouts on potatoes and delaying ripening of fruits.

The concern is that irradiation changes the chemistry of the food, producing new compounds called radiolytic products (RP). Most of the RPs are naturally present in foods, up to 90 percent, but a small number are unique. Although the FDA has approved the process, many consumer groups have continued to protest, and research on the safety of RP continues.

Raffinose: A naturally occurring compound found in sugar beets, roots, cottonseed, and molasses. Humans can't break it down, and after it travels to the colon, bacteria ferment raffinose, causing gas and other intestinal symptoms (see *fiber*).

Saponins: Compounds found in grapes, legumes, and soybeans which interfere with DNA reproduction and may prevent cancer cell multiplication. In addition, studies show that they may also interfere with cholesterol absorption. A negative effect may include interference with the absorption of fat soluble vitamins.

Short-Chain Fatty Acids (SCFA): Fatty acids (see *fatty acids*) containing less than six carbons; they have less calories than longer fatty acids. Foods contain small amounts, and most SCFA in the human body arise from bacteria in the colon-digesting fiber. Soluble fiber is the best substrate for bacteria to make these fatty acids. Higher levels of SCFA act as a laxative and cause diarrhea. Researchers are studying SCFA for potential health benefits, especially in preventing colon cancer.

Solanine: A toxic compound present in potato peels and sprouts. The compound forms in potatoes when the vegetables are stored improperly, exposing them to light and temperature extremes. Cooking temperatures don't destroy solanine, but most of the compound is contained in the peel, which is often discarded. Small amounts of solanine are harmless, but at high intakes it exerts a narcoticlike effect, producing symptoms of headache, abdominal pain, vomiting, diarrhea, and fever. In addition, it causes neurologic symptoms including apathy, confusion, and hallucinations. Green spots on potatoes indicate high concentrations of solanine.

Sorbitol: A sugar alcohol used as an alternative sweetener. It has the same caloric value as sugar, but the body absorbs it more slowly, so it was thought to be useful for people with diabetes. However, the latest recommendations from the American Diabetes Association state that alternative sweeteners do not offer special advantages over sugar in maintaining blood glucose control over time. High intakes of sorbitol have caused gastrointestinal problems in some people.

Starch (food starches as additives): Polysaccharides in the carbohydrate category of nutrients. Starches exist in two forms, amylopectin and amylose. The latter is a chain of up to 2,000 basic sugar units, glucose, while the amylopectin consists of a branched molecule with up to several thousand glucose units. Most starches contain a mixture of both, the proportion varying with the type of starch. As food additives, a variety of starch compounds confer important functional properties on food, making possible new and innovative products.

In the food industry, common starches used include potato, corn, rice, wheat, and tapioca. In the past, deciding which starch to use was usually dependent on the country in which the product was made and its staple grain. More recently, however, food technologists have uncovered the unique properties which various starch sources bestow on the product, so that the use determines the source.

An important aspect of starch sources, aside from the proportions of amylopectin and amylose, is the size and shape of the individual starch granules. They can either be tightly packed or more loosely layered. In addition, the molecules of amylopectin and amylose mingle via hydrogen bonding to form bundles called micelles. The micelles keep the granules connected and stable to prevent the individual starch molecules from dissolving.

Some of the different functional properties of starches include adhesion, binding, film forming, water-holding, gelling, and thickening. Depending on what the finished product is to be, the desired functional property will be sought and its associated starch source. As an example, if the finished product is to be frozen, the water-holding capacity of the starch will be most important to maintain texture and mouthfeel. Some typical foods in which various starches are used include instant mixes, soups, frozen foods, and salad dressings. Many new low-fat foods owe the reduction in fat to starch. As new products are continually developed, many more uses can be expected of designer starches.

Sulfites: Compounds which are oxides of the mineral sulfur and have wide applications in the food industry. Some of these applications include sanitizing food containers and equipment, inhibiting wine and beer fermentation, and preserving color and flavor, and preventing spoilage in the following foods: seafood, dried and fresh fruits, and fresh vegetables. Sulfites were widely used by restaurants to keep fruits and vegetables fresh in salad bars. However, the FDA banned this use of sulfites and now requires the compounds to be included on food labels after reports of several deaths from severe allergic reactions. The reactions typically involved people with asthma who experienced weakness, wheezing, and chest tightness. On food labels, sulfites appear as sulfur dioxide, sodium sulfite, sodium bisulfite, potassium bisulfite, sodium metabisulfite, and potassium metabisulfite.

Tannins: Polyphenol compounds present in tea, coffee, nuts, and some fruits and vegetables. Tannins can interfere with the absorption of essential trace minerals, especially iron. They are of current interest to researchers who have recognized their antioxidant ability, which may protect against diseases such as cancer and heart disease.

Tartrazine: Chemical name for yellow color FD&C Yellow No. 5, which is currently FDA approved for use in foods, drugs, and cosmetics (see *food coloring agents*). Some individuals may be allergic to tartrazine, triggering breathing difficulties and bronchial asthma.

Taurine: A sulfur-containing amino acid which is not one of the essential amino acids. In humans, taurine is present in most cells and concentrated in the fetal nervous system, muscles, and platelets, and occurs in bile. Taurine appears to be involved in regulating many activities such as heartbeat, membrane integrity, and platelet aggregation. The body can make taurine from methionine and cysteine, and the diet provides a good supply of the amino acid. The best sources include meat and fish, with virtually none in plant foods. Although it's not deemed essential yet, some studies show that under certain conditions, a dietary source may be essential. Because researchers had reported that premature infants required taurine, infant formulas now contain it.

Tryptophan: An essential amino acid needed for tissue synthesis and a precursor for the neurotransmitter serotonin and the B vitamin niacin. Eating carbohydrate foods along with a source of tryptophan can cause drowsiness by increasing serotonin production. About nine years ago, tryptophan supplements from Japan caused a mysterious ailment called eosinophilia myalgia syndrome that resulted in several deaths. After this, the FDA recalled all products containing tryptophan.

Tyramine: An amine compound present in many foods, which produces similar physiologic effects as epinephrine (adrenalin).

People who use drugs called monoamine oxidase inhibitors (MAO inhibitors) must avoid foods containing tyramine because of a potential deadly effect. The enzyme, monoamine oxidase, normally breaks down tyramine, but MAO inhibitors prevent this from occurring. Consequently, tyramine accumulates and can cause severe hypertension, possibly even a stroke. Foods containing tyramine are usually products of bacterial fermentation and include ale and beer, red wines, liqueurs, aged and processed cheeses, pickled herring and salted dried fish, and dry sausages such as salami, pepperoni, and bologna. Other foods containing tyramine include legumes, liver, meat extracts, and brewer's yeast.

Umami: A recently discovered fifth human taste in addition to sweet, sour, salty, and bitter. Although food technologists have been stimulating umami for years with the addition of monosodium glutamate (MSG) to commercial foods, it wasn't clear why this compound enhances flavor. Researchers recently reported that certain taste buds in the mouths of animals react only to MSG, a food additive which many people are surprised to learn occurs naturally in virtually all foods.

The name for this newfound taste is a Japanese word (pronounced oo-MOM-ee) and roughly translates to "delicious." The closest description of umami's taste is that it imparts a meatlike flavor. The food industry has long capitalized on umami by adding MSG to snacks and meals which, by enhancing flavor, increases one's appetite for more of the product. MSG, the salt form of the amino acid glutamate, has repeatedly come under fire for a variety of alleged ill effects, but the FDA cleared the compound's reputation in 1995 by stating that MSG was safe.

Foods high in MSG, such as tomatoes, grapefruit, potatoes, mushrooms, and parmesan cheese, stimulate the umami taste buds, which send electrical impulses to the brain. The brain, in turn, sends signals to increase intake of the food item. The average person has 2,000 to 5,000 taste buds, although some people may have as many as 10,000 and, along with the extra taste buds, a heightened sense of taste. The studies were conducted with rats, but taste buds in essentially all animals are similar to those of humans.

Nutritionists are hopeful that further studies may provide the answers to stimulating taste buds and therefore appetite in people whose food intake is compromised. This would particularly benefit many elderly people with poor appetites, as well as people with diseases such as cancer in which poor appetite and loss of taste are common problems, leading to malnutrition.

Whey: The liquid that remains after the curd and cream are separated and removed from milk which has been coagulated in order to make products such as cheese. Nutritionally, it contains most of the lactose from the milk and some water soluble nutrients, but almost none of the protein and fat. Most people think of Little Miss Muffet when they see the word *whey* on food labels, and may wonder why it's in their frozen pizza. Whey has a growing list of uses in the food industry, and food product designers anticipate many more in the future.

In the not too distant past of human history, whey was considered a waste product. Early cheesemakers noticed that after coagulating milk, they had the desired curd and cream and a somewhat clear liquid with no apparent use. This waste product notion was reinforced after chemical analysis determined that whey contained most of the lactose of the whole milk, but little protein and no fat.

As food science advanced, separation technology emerged, enabling the isolation of whey protein and assuring its place in the food industry. Some of the more interesting uses include its addition to reduced-fat versions of foods such as hamburgers or cheesecake. It is also desirable because of its low flavor profile.

Even with its vast array of current uses and remarkable potential in designing future foods, half of the whey produced in the United States is discarded. The main problem is the costs involved in the necessary separation technology, which is beyond many smaller manufacturers. This problem is bypassed by manufacturers who produce and use their own whey.

One of the most common forms is dried whole whey, which is processed without requiring sophisticated equipment, yielding 75 percent lactose and 12 percent protein. Dried whey continues to be used in products such as sauces, cheese breads, and other baked goods, to which it imparts dairy flavor. However, the protein content is not high enough to be used for fortification, which food designers see as the wave of the future in nutraceutical products. Manufacturers use the following terms: whey protein concentrate, whey protein isolate, dried whey, and total milk protein (contains both whey and casein).

Resources on the World Wide Web

T he following list pulls together a variety of online resources, which provide information and education for consumers on nutrition and health issues. The list is not exhaustive and doesn't imply support of the content. Remember that World Wide Web addresses (URLs) can change, so if you can't access a particular site using the URL listed, try doing a search with the group's name. One of the sites listed is Wayne State University, and you can access this site for nutrition information, as well as e-mail me with questions.

Government Agencies

Links to government agencies, including those related to food safety and health
http://www.consumer.gov

Food and Drug Administration Consumer Publication
http://www.fda.gov/fdac/fdachtml.html

A Gateway for Consumer Health Information from the Government
http://www.healthfinder.gov

USDA Food Composition Tables
http://www.nal.usda.gov/fnic/food comp/

World Health Organization
http://www.who.ch

Centers for Disease Control and Prevention
http://www.cdc.gov

From U.S. Dept. of Agriculture, School Meals Program
http://schoolmeals.nal.usda.gov:8001

National Institutes of Health Homepage
http://www.nih.gov/

National Cancer Institute
http://www.nci.nih

U.S. Dept. of Agriculture Center for Nutrition Policy and Promotion
http://www.usda.gov/fcs/cnpp

U.S. Dept. of Health and Human Services
http://www.os.dhhs.gov

Public Access to MedLine
http://www.ncbi.nlm.nih.gov

Industry and Trade Groups

News and info on fat-free eating and products
http://www.fatfree.com/

Food Information Council
http://www.crcpress.com/fcn/titlepg.htm

National Soyfoods Directory
http://soyfoods.com

Nonprofit Organizations

American Diabetes Association
http://www.diabetes.org

American Heart Association
http://www.amhrt.org

Biotechnology Information Center
http://www.inform.umd.edu:8080/EdRes/Topic/AgrEnv/Biotech

Dietetics Online
http://www.dietetics.com

National Council Against Health Fraud's home page
http://www.primenet.com/~ncahf/

The Vegetarian Resource Group
http://www.vrg.org

The International Food Information Council
http://ificinfo.health.org/

Quackwatch, Information About Health Fraud
http://www.qwackwatch.com

Food Allergy Network
http://www.foodallergy.org/index.html

Professional Associations and Journals

**American Association of Family Physicians; America's
Housecall Network**
http://www.housecall.com

The American Dietetics Association
http://www.eatright.org

American Medical Association (AMA)
http://www.ama-assn.org/journals/most/recent/issues/jama/toc.htm

American Public Health Association
http://www.apha.org

American Society for Clinical Nutrition
http://www.faseb.org/ascn

New England Journal of Medicine
http://www.nejm.org

Universities

University of Michigan Medical Center
http://www.med.umich.edu

Tulane University Medical Center
http://www.mcl.tulane.edu

University of Wisconsin, InfoLink
http://www.biostat.wisc.edu

Dietary Approaches to Stop Hypertension
http://www.dash.bwh.harvard.edu

University of Minnesota Food Science and Nutrition
http://fscn1.fsci.umn.edu/

OncoLink
http://cancer.med.upenn.edu/

Wayne State University Nutrition and Food Science Department
http://www.science.wayne.edu/~nfs

Bibliography

Claudio, Virginia S., and Rosalinda T. Lagua. *Nutrition and Diet Therapy Dictionary.* New York: Van Nostrand Reinhold, 1991.

Escott-Stump, Sylvia. *Nutrition and Diagnosis-Related Care.* Baltimore: Williams & Wilkins, 1997.

Mahan, Kathleen L., and Sylvia Escott-Stump. *Krause's Food, Nutrition, & Diet Therapy.* Philadelphia: W. B. Saunders Company, 1996.

Pennington, Jean A. T. *Bowes and Church's Food Values of Portions Commonly Used.* Philadelphia: J. B. Lippincott Company, 1994.

Recommended Dietary Allowances, 10th ed. Washington, D.C.: National Academy Press, 1989.

Shils, Maurice E., James A. Olson, and Moshe Shike. *Modern Nutrition in Health and Disease.* Philadelphia: Lea & Febiger, 1994.

"The Surgeon General's Report on Nutrition and Health." Washington, D.C.: U.S. Government Printing Office, 1988.

Whitney, Eleanor N., Corinne B. Cataldo, and Sharon R. Rolfes. *Understanding Normal and Clinical Nutrition.* Belmont, Calif.: Wadsworth Publishing Company, 1998.

Zeman, Frances J., and Denise M. Ney. *Applications in Medical Nutrition Therapy.* Englewood Cliffs, N.J.: Prentice-Hall, Inc., 1996.

Index